General Practice Revisited

Ann Cartwright
and Robert Anderson
Institute for Social Studies
in Medical Care

General Practice Revisited

A Second Study of Patients and Their Doctors

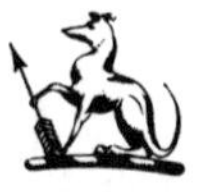

TAVISTOCK PUBLICATIONS

First published in 1981 by
Tavistock Publications Ltd
11 New Fetter Lane, London EC4P 4EE
Published in the USA by
Tavistock Publications
in association with Methuen, Inc.
733 Third Avenue, New York, NY 10017

Printed in Great Britain at the
University Press, Cambridge

British Library Cataloguing in Publication data

Cartwright, Ann
General practice revisited.
1. Family medicine – England – History
– 20th century
I. Title *II. Anderson, Robert,* b. 1944
362. 1' 0425 *R729.5.G4* *80–41126*

ISBN 0–422–77360–3

Contents

Foreword

In our study of patients and their doctors in 1977 we collected a great deal of data. Some are comparable with data collected in 1964; other material concentrated on more recent developments.In making decisions about what questions to ask and which analyses to make we have been concerned with various propositions about trends in primary care and with ideas about its organization and about the relationship between patients and doctors. Sometimes we have discussed the reasoning behind the analyses, but often it is implied rather than stated directly. Our basic aim has been to describe the experiences and views of both patients and their doctors in 1977 and, where relevant, to show how these have changed since 1964.

The book is written for people concerned with information about the functioning of our primary care system. Many of these people will have their own ideas about what is happening and will want to see whether our data support their theories or not.

We have aimed at presenting our data clearly and succinctly within a simple framework. We have placed our results within the context of the changes that took place between the two surveys but have not tried to write a systematic or comprehensive account of the relevant political, legal, or social changes in that period. Such accounts are available elsewhere (Honigsbaum 1979; Hicks 1976; Watkin 1975).*

* References are given in full at the end of the book.

Having decided to do this study, to collect these data and to analyse them in a particular way, it would not be appropriate just to present our results and leave others to interpret them. We have expressed our views about the changes, and the lack of change, and, particularly in the last chapter, we have discussed what we see as the main implications of our findings.

Hampstead
February 1980

ANN CARTWRIGHT
ROBERT ANDERSON

Acknowledgements

We are very grateful to the many people who helped and contributed to this study:

the patients and their doctors who gave up their time and answered our many questions;

the interviewers, especially Hillary Gellman and the late Muriel Toney, who supervised;

the coders: Andy Britton, Margaret Hall, Richard Mond, and Ming Moseley-Williams;

Christopher Smith who checked our figures and statements and contributed to the appendices;

Alison Venning who prepared the data for analysis and helped in many other ways;

Janet Ball and Michele Becker who typed the documents and gave administrative support; and Moira Purves and Irene Browne who prepared this report;

other colleagues at the Institute for Social Studies in Medical Care, most notably Louise Holland who helped in the administration of the fieldwork, and Ann Bowling and Madeleine Simms who made helpful comments;

members of the Institute's Advisory Committee, who supported and advised at various stages: Abe Adelstein, Tony Alment, Val Beral, Vera Carstairs, May Clarke, Geoffrey Hawthorn, Austin

Heady, Margot Jefferys, Joyce Leeson, John McEwan, David Morrell, and Martin Richards;

Joan Deane and Dorothy Hills who punched the cards;

Sheila Gray and David Cable at the Office of Population Censuses and Surveys, and Mr Nickless at the DHSS for their time and resources;

the DHSS which funded the study and particularly Arthur Forsdick, Doreen Rothman, and Marguerite Smith;

the Royal College of General Practitioners and General Medical Services Committee which expressed support for the study, and Janet Smith who prepared data on College membership;

the Department of Community Medicine at Manchester University which gave hospitality;

people who helped in various other ways, including Patsy Bailey, Ron Blunden, Gwen Cartwright, Ruth Cooperstock, Karen Dunnell, David Fruin, Andrew Herxheimer, John Horder, Geoff Horton, Geoffrey Marsh, Jack Norell, Mims Orleans, Eric Roughley, Alwyn Smith, Peter Sowerby, Margaret Stacey, and Jasper Woodcock.

1 Introduction

In 1964 when an earlier study, *Patients and their doctors* (Cartwright 1967) was carried out, the future of general practice was being questioned by some critics who held that the increasing specialization of medical care made the generalist redundant. Defenders reasoned that: 'The more complex medicine becomes, the stronger are the reasons why everyone should have a personal doctor who will take continuous responsibility for him, and, knowing how he lives, will keep things in proportion – protecting him, if need be, from the zealous specialist' (Fox 1960). By 1977, when the more recent study was done, the argument was no longer about whether general practice should survive but on how it should develop. There were discussions about the importance of team care, about the advantages and disadvantages of health centres, about the role of home visiting, and about the form and content of education for general practice. Renewed confidence in general practice appeared to be related to changes in conditions of work, to changes in education and influence, and to 'economic difficulties and their effects on high-cost, high-technology hospital medicine' which made it 'increasingly evident that no nation (could) afford rapid and continuing expansion of the practice of this type of medicine, and that the comparatively lower-cost, lower-technology medicine practised in primary care must expand to treat yet more diseases in the community' (Fry 1977: xii).

The main origins of the changes in conditions of work and education are listed in *Table 1.*

Table 1 Main origins of change 1964–77

Amendment of general practitioners' terms of service in 1966 (The GP's Charter): involving pay increases; extra payments for seniority, group practice, out of hours work, and work in designated areas; encouraged employment of ancillary staff.
Establishment of General Practice Finance Corporation in 1967: provided loans for general practitioners to finance new practice premises and remodel old ones.
Granting of Royal status to the College of General Practitioners in 1967: the recognition and enhancement of its increasing influence.
The Health Services and Public Health Act 1968: extended the spheres of action of nurses, health visitors, and midwives in the community.
Royal Commission on Medical Education 1968: recognized general practice as a speciality in its own right, recommended vocational training of general practitioners; led to the introduction of a three-year post-graduate training for doctors going into general practice, to the development of post-graduate medical centres all over the country, and to the establishment of departments of general practice in most medical schools.
Local Authority Social Services Act, 1970: the establishment of unified social service departments in each major local authority perpetuating and accentuating the administrative division between health and social services.
Report on the Organisation of Group Practice 1971: rejected the decentralization of laboratory and X-ray services, recommended that general practitioners should be given full access to these facilities at the district hospital.
The reorganization of the National Health Service in 1974: consultants and general practitioners brought together in management and in planning in the hope that this would lead to closer understanding and cooperation between them.

Watkin (1977: 215–16) sums up: 'If in 1963 general practitioners still saw themselves as the Cinderellas of the medical profession, by the early 1970s their position was clearly a much more comfortable one, both in financial terms and in terms of professional standing and self-esteem'.

But with all the changes there had been little attempt to assess their effects on either patients or doctors. Our aim is to fill part of this gap by looking at the views and experiences of both patients and doctors in 1977 and, where relevant, comparing our findings with those of the earlier, 1964, study.

Aims

As in 1964 our aim is to describe the care given by the general practitioner service and the attitudes of patients and doctors to this care. Again there are obvious limitations to our approach. No attempt is made to assess the clinical skills and judgements of the doctors. But if clinical expertise is to be used effectively the doctor must be accessible to the patients who need these skills. A good patient-doctor relationship is a prerequisite for much good medical care. Our problem is to assess the relationships in useful and appropriate terms since the nature of people's relationships with their general practitioner varies so widely. Some may hardly know their doctor, others may depend on him or her to such an extent that they may be unwilling to discuss their relationship. It may have been that on occasion neither patients nor doctors answered our questions fully, frankly, or accurately. These are the inevitable hazards of such studies. We try to minimize the shortcomings but we cannot hope to eliminate them entirely. A further complication arises when we make comparisons over time, since people's standards and expectations change. So changes in the level of criticism have to be interpreted with care and may not reflect improvements or deteriorations in the services.

By looking at the effect of some of the recent changes in the form and content of general practice the study aims to identify possible developments which will foster mutual understanding between patients and doctors and encourage the appropriate use of resources.

Methods

The study was done in twenty parliamentary constituencies in England and Wales. They were selected after stratification with probability proportional to the number of electors. Further details of the way this was done and of the study areas appear in Appendix I. In each area a random sample of fifty people were chosen from the electoral register, which had been published in February 1977. Eight hundred and thirty-six people out of the 1,000 selected were successfully interviewed in their own homes between April and July

1977. This is our sample of patients or potential patients. More information about the selection and response of patients appears in Appendix II. Reasons for our failure to interview all the people are shown in *Table 2.* Most of the interviews, 73%, lasted between one and two hours; only 7% were shorter, but 20% were longer. A structured questionnaire was used, a copy of which may be obtained from the Institute for Social Studies in Medical Care.*

Those who were interviewed were asked for the name and address of the general practitioner whose NHS list they were on. Sixteen, 2%, were not on the list of an NHS doctor who they would consult if they were ill but five of these had a private doctor whose name and address they gave us.** We were unable to trace the doctors of six patients because the information proved inadequate. The other 819 patients gave us the names of 543 different doctors. Ninety one per cent of these patients gave us the name of the doctor whose list they were on, the other 9% gave us the names of doctors in the same practice who they felt they knew better and regarded as their doctor. These doctors were sent a letter and a postal questionnaire and after two reminders 365, 67%, returned a completed questionnaire. This is our sample of general practitioners.

Table 2 Patients' response

Interviewed	836
Refusal	99
Died	10
Unable to contact – never in	6
– moved	39
Too ill, deaf, or other reason	10
Total	1,000

The response rate among patients was similar to that on the 1964 study but both studies depend on the completeness of the electoral register for their representativeness. People who, for any reason, are not on the register in the area where they are now living will not generally be represented, so the study will not give a picture of the

* 14 South Hill Park, London, NW3 2SB. There will be a charge for photocopying when supplies run out.

** The others are discussed in more detail in Appendix VII.

problems of mobile people who have difficulty finding a doctor who will accept them on his or her NHS list. However the age, sex, and marital status distributions of our sample of patients are similar to that of the adult population in England and Wales (Central Statistical Office 1978).

Among general practitioners the response rate fell from 76% in 1964 to 67% in 1977. Comparisons using data from the Department of Health and Social Security do not show any significant variation* in the response rate this time with age, sex, or size of partnership, but those with licentiate qualifications only were less likely to reply (55% of them did so, compared with 70% of those with other qualifications) and those who qualified in India, Pakistan, Bangladesh, or Sri Lanka (subsequently referred to as Asians) were also less likely to respond (53% against 69% of doctors who qualified elsewhere). Members of the Royal College of General Practitioners and appointed general practitioner trainers had comparatively high response rates of 78% and 84% respectively.

In addition to data from the DHSS we also have information from patients so it is possible to compare patients' attitudes to doctors who participated and to those who failed to respond. They had similar reactions to the two groups. So although the low response rate from general practitioners is a cause for concern the bias does not seem to be great.

Another source of bias in the sample of general practitioners is that the chance of a doctor being asked to participate in the inquiry is related to the number of patients – that is, to the people who regarded him or her as their doctor. For many purposes this built-in bias is a reasonable one. From the point of view of the service given to all patients, a doctor who has twice as many patients as another doctor is twice as important. Many of the analyses are therefore made on the sample of patients' doctors, with doctors reported by two patients included twice, by three patients three times, etc.

For analyses which involve doctors only – not patients – the unweighted sample of doctors is used although it is not a strictly random sample – the chance of being included at all is related in some way, but not directly, to a doctor's number of patients. But, as is shown in Appendix III, the effect of this bias is relatively small

* In general, attention is not drawn to differences which might have occurred by chance five or more times in 100. A discussion of statistical significance and sampling errors appears in Appendix IV.

even with things strongly related to doctors' estimates of the number of patients they looked after.

The book

In the main part of the book we deal with changes and developments in general practice and relate these to the experiences and attitudes of both patients and doctors.

We start by looking at the setting in which general practice is carried out, particularly at partnerships, the continuity of care, accessibility, family care, and emergency arrangements, and then go on to look at changes in the frequency and nature of doctor-patient contacts. After that we take a look at health centres – the doctors who work in them, the way they work and their perceptions of the advantages and disadvantages of health centres. And of course we see how patients feel about them. In the following chapter we consider the other members of the primary care team; particularly receptionists, nurses, and social workers, and subsequently the relationship between hospitals and general practitioners is examined. In a chapter on variations between doctors we consider their age, sex, training, and country of qualification; while in the chapter on variations between patients the characteristics we look at are age, sex, and social class. In a final chapter we summarize our findings and review their implications.

Before starting on these analyses it is appropriate to consider the general level of patients' and doctors' satisfactions and criticisms so that in looking at their comments on specific issues we can put them in perspective.

Patients' views and criticisms

'Behind the satisfaction of most patients there lies an uncritical acceptance and lack of discrimination which is conducive to stagnation and apathy.' This was one of the conclusions of the 1964 study. Was the same true thirteen years later?

In general, both patients and doctors in 1977 thought that patients were more rather than less likely to question whether the doctor was right than they were ten years ago: 30% of patients aged 25 or more thought this about themselves, 57% of doctors who had been in general practice for two years or more thought this about their patients.* The fact that rather more doctors than patients perceived a change is to be expected as patients were responding only about themselves, doctors about trends among their patients. In addition, 72% of doctors thought their patients were more knowledgeable about health matters now. (Over half the patients, 53%, felt their knowledge of health matters was greater than it had been ten years earlier but of course few, 1%, thought it was less.) There was clear agreement between the two groups about the direction of change, and in our view the change is an encouraging one: to more knowledgeable and less passive patients.

Has there been a change in the level of patients' criticisms? In both studies patients were asked whether they felt their doctor was 'good' or 'not so good' about a series of things. Their replies are shown in *Table 3*.

Table 3 Proportion of patients who were critical of various aspects of their general practitioner care on the two studies

	1964	*1977*
*Proportion who felt their doctor was 'not so good' about:**		
Having well-equipped up-to-date surgery	18% (1108)	19% (684)
Having a pleasant comfortable waiting room	24% (1194)	30% (711)
Always visiting when asked	3% (1168)	13% (569)
Sending people to hospital as soon as necessary	4% (963)	8% (552)
Keeping people waiting in waiting room	17% (1069)	21% (671)
Examining people carefully and thoroughly	6% (1135)	13% (669)
Only sending people to hospital when necessary	2% (859)	3% (560)
Taking time and not hurrying you	6% (1237)	14% (712)
Listening to what you say	3% (1260)	7% (715)
Explaining things to you fully	16% (1168)	23% (692)

* The proportion who said their doctor was 'not so good' out of those who said he/she was either 'good' or 'not so good' has been used. Those who said they did not know or made some other comment have been excluded, since there were different criteria for asking the question on the two studies. Figures in brackets are the numbers on which the percentages are based (= 100%).

* Doctors who had been in general practice for between two and ten years were asked about changes during this period, those who had been in for longer were asked about changes in the last ten years.

On eight of the ten criteria patients were more critical in the later survey. (The exceptions were 'having a well-equipped up-to-date surgery' and 'only sending people to hospital when necessary' for neither of which was there a significant change in the proportion who were critical.) Part of the increase in criticism almost certainly stems from higher expectations and standards, so can be seen as a positive rather than a negative change. For instance we will show that waiting times have shortened somewhat. And while there was a marked increase in the proportion of patients who were critical of their doctors for not explaining things, among the patients aged 25 or more who were interviewed in 1977, 29% thought their doctor explained things more fully than he or she (or the doctor they had then) had done ten years previously, while 10% thought he or she explained less. Even among those who thought their doctor was better now about explaining things, 14% were still critical of the way he or she did so.

There was a four-fold increase in the proportion who were critical of their doctor about visiting and in addition the proportion who did not categorize their doctor as either good or not so good about visiting increased from 16% in 1964 to 32%. This was probably because of their lack of experience over this on the later study, while the increase in criticism is almost certainly attributable to a greater unwillingness among doctors to visit patients at home. This is discussed in Chapter 3.

Expression of criticism is one indication of changing views and experiences: action is another. In 1964 and 1977 similar proportions of patients, a third, had changed their doctor in the five years before the interview, and in both studies nine-tenths of the changes occurred either because the patient moved or the doctor retired, moved, or died. Only a small proportion of patients had changed because they were dissatisfied with their doctor but the proportion of changes attributed to this had if anything decreased from 8% in 1964 to 4% in 1977. Changes in actions also need to be interpreted with care. It could be that with the increase in partnerships more patients can select a doctor, within the practice, who suits them, so that fewer want to change (see Aylett 1976). Another possibility is that patients now see it as more difficult to find a doctor in another practice who would accept them if they wanted to change because they felt critical of their doctor. The proportion of patients who felt their doctor was the only reasonably accessible doctor, or group of doctors, had increased from 14% in 1964 to 19% in 1977. This is one indication that they felt their choice was more limited in 1977. In both studies 10% of patients said they had thought of changing their present doctor.

Another index of dissatisfaction is turning to private instead of National Health Service care, but of course this possibility is only open to those who can afford it. In both 1964 and 1977 less than 1% of people interviewed did not have a National Health Service doctor but said they had a regular private one who they had consulted before and would consult again if they were ill. In 1964, 2% of those with an NHS doctor said they had consulted a private doctor in the last twelve months; in 1977 this proportion was 3% but less than 1% had consulted a general practitioner privately, 2% had seen a specialist consultant.*

In this more recent study three of the twenty-eight who had consulted a doctor privately or who had a private general practitioner were covered under an insurance scheme, that is less than half of a per cent of all patients. But seventy other patients, that is 8% of the sample, said they had some insurance to cover private medical care. Other data suggest that in 1977 4% of the population in the United Kingdom were insured under private medical insurance, but this is based on the total population and includes children (Central Statistical Office 1979). An earlier study (Gray and Cartwright 1953) found 2% of people were using or would use private general practitioner care only and another 2% used both NHS and private primary care.

Although there is the possibility that people who have opted out of the National Health Service may be less willing to participate in studies of medical care, it is clear that the great majority of people rely on the National Health Service for all their primary health care.

To sum up, the changes so far are generally encouraging. There is no evidence that more patients are changing or thinking of changing their doctor because they are dissatisfied with the care they are receiving. At the same time more patients are expressing criticisms of certain aspects of their care. Much of this increase appears to stem from higher expectations and a greater willingness to express criticisms of a service which the great majority value highly. In 1977 nine-tenths of patients described themselves as 'very

* For further discussion of private patients see Appendix VII.

satisfied' or 'satisfied' with the care they had received from their doctor. But from the patients' point of view the service has clearly deteriorated in one respect – the willingness of doctors to visit people in their homes.

Doctors' views and criticisms

Nineteen sixty-four, when the earlier study was carried out, was two years before the introduction of the Family Doctor's Charter (1966). Morale in general practice was thought to be low, particularly in relation to pay and conditions of work. However, general practitioners' assessments of the extent to which they enjoyed their work were similar on the two studies *(Table 4)*.

Table 4 General practitioners' enjoyment of their work

	1964	*1977*
	%	%
On the whole enjoys general practice:		
Very much	52	55
Moderately	37	36
Not very much	9	7
Not at all	2	1
Other comment	—	1
*Number of general practitioners (= 100%)**	414	365

* A small proportion for whom inadequate information was obtained have been excluded from this and later tables when calculating percentages.

There were some changes in the aspects of their work that they enjoyed *(Table 5)*. Although a lower proportion of those on the later study said they enjoyed all of it there were increases in the proportion who mentioned their freedom and independence, and the variety of the work, and in the small proportion who said they enjoyed treating people with medical problems. There were some changes in the way the responses were classified which makes it impossible to compare the proportion who said they enjoyed visiting people at home or being a family doctor.

It is less easy to make straightforward comparisons over what doctors found frustrating *(Table 6)*.However, there has been an increase in the proportion complaining about overwork – this in

Table 5 What general practitioners enjoyed about their work

1964			*1977*
	%	%	
Patients, people, human beings, and personal contact, friend of family, social contact	46	45	People: contact with people and humanity, knowing people over time, establishing relationships with patients, trust, giving continuous, ongoing care
Variety, diversity (of people or diseases or unspecified)	18	25	Variety, diversity (of people or diseases or unspecified), unpredictability
Freedom/independence – professional or from supervision, to diagnose and/or treat	10	26	Freedom/independence: complete responsibility for diagnosis and/or treatment, freedom to manage and organise own work, being own master
Being a help to others, doing some good, curing people, relieving suffering	17	16	Being a help to others, doing some good, relieving suffering, curing people, seeing good results of my work, doing useful job
Visiting people, going into people's homes	4	18	Being a family doctor, knowing family and their medical/social environment, visiting people in their homes
Diagnosis	7	8	Diagnosis: interpreting/solving problems
Appreciation	4	4	Appreciation: feeling your good work is recognised by others in the community
Really sick, genuine acute cases	4	8	Clinical medicine: treating people with (genuine) medical problems
All of it – but nothing specified	9	3	All of it – but nothing specified
Nothing	4	2	Nothing – or very little
Others	22	15	Others
Number of doctors (= 100%)	398	340	

Table 6 What general practitioners found frustrating about their work

1964	%			%	*1977*
Trivial conditions, minor complaints, unnecessary consultations	34	48		40	Patients: excessive demands, abuse, consulting with minor or inappropriate conditions, negative attitudes of patients/public, lack of self-reliance, being called out unnecessarily, general criticisms of patients
Patients – some or all – any comment which was directly critical of patients	25				
Too many patients, inadequate time to do work properly, pressure of work	20			27	Overworked: too many consultations, volume of work because too many patients, inadequate time to do work properly
Clerical work/forms/certificates	18			17	Administration (personal): clerical work, certification, committee work, form-filling, anxieties about maintenance of premises
Late calls or calls at wrong times	11	25		8	Lack of leisure/free time: always being on call, holidays night calls, uncertainty of times of work
Inadequate leisure, free time, holidays, hours of work	10				
Being tired, always on call, never left in peace	5				
Pay	12			9	Remuneration: method or amount of, way in which it works against good/better medical practice
			39	9	Outside interference: government/administrators, general bureaucracy, management
Others	37			20	Hospital, social, and ancillary services
				3	Limitations of self or of medicine
				12	Other
Nothing	2			5	Nothing
Number of doctors (= 100%)	408			356	

spite of the increase in ancillary services and the decrease in home visiting. It may be that doctors' expectations about workloads have changed. Another possibility is that the presence of partners and ancillary workers makes general practitioners more aware of other needs.

The most marked change was the drop in the proportion complaining about late calls, inadequate leisure, and being tied. The increase in deputizing services and partnerships would appear to have had a very positive effect in this respect.

There was no decline in the proportion reporting that they found clerical work and other administrative tasks frustrating.

Although a lower proportion of doctors in 1977 than in 1964 were spontaneously critical of their patients or mentioned consultations for trivial conditions as one of the things they found frustrating, there was no difference in the proportion of their surgery consultations which they felt were for trivial, inappropriate, or unnecessary reasons. In both studies the estimated average was a third of all consultations. The distributions are in *Table 7.*

Table 7 Trivial consultations

	1964	*1977*
Proportion of surgery consultations doctors estimate are for reasons they feel to be trivial, unnecessary, or inappropriate	%	%
90% or more	2	1
75% but less than 90%	5	7
50% but less than 75%	19	16
25% but less than 50%	30	26
10% but less than 25%	29	31
Less than 10%	15	19
Number of general practitioners (=100%)	420	359

The nature of 'trivial' consultations and the characteristics of doctors who regard different proportions of their consultations as falling into this category will be examined in later chapters.

A lack of change in doctors' attitudes to and enjoyment of their work is the main finding so far.

2 The setting

In this chapter we discuss some of the changes in the ways in which general practitioners organize their work which followed the legislative and administrative measures described in the last chapter. One development has been the increase in partnerships and the impact of this on both patients and doctors is examined first. Other organizational changes such as the increase in appointment systems are also considered as are the implications of these changes for continuity of care, for accessibility, and for family care. Finally changes in arrangements for night calls and in equipment at the practice are described.

Partnerships – the patient's perspective

The proportion of patients who thought their doctor worked on his own fell from 19% in 1964 to 12% in 1977, and the proportion who said he worked with just one other doctor also dropped from 34% to 19%.* But this change was not accompanied by an increase in the proportion who said they preferred a doctor who worked in

* When information was available from both patients and doctors it tallied in terms of whether the practice was single handed or not in 96% of instances. But in terms of the precise number of doctors working together agreement was less good, and tallied in only 67% of cases. When considering the views of patients we have taken their statements about the size of partnerships, but when we consider the viewpoint of the doctors we have taken their statements.

partnership. In 1977, 31% said they preferred a doctor who worked on his own, 41% one in a partnership, and 28% thought it did not matter – no change in the ratio between the first two proportions from 1964 but a decrease in the proportion who felt it did not matter, which was 36% in the earlier study. So among those with a preference for a single-handed doctor the proportion who had a doctor who worked on his own had fallen from 40% in 1964 to 25% in 1977. On both studies the proportion expressing a preference for what they had was higher for those with a doctor who worked on his own than for those whose doctor worked with others (see *Table 8*).

Table 8 Patients' preferences for a single-handed doctor or one in a partnership

	Proportion preferring what they have			
	1964		*1977*	
Those with:				
Doctor on own	57%	(251)	65%	(95)
Doctor in partnership	42%	(1050)	45%	(699)
All patients	45%	(1301)	47%	(794)

Figures in brackets are numbers on which percentages are based (= *100%*).

Overall the proportion who preferred what they had was similar on the two studies, largely because fewer people on the more recent study felt it did not matter. However the proportion preferring what they did *not* have (in terms of a partnership or single-handed doctor) had increased from 19% to 25%.

In 1964 older patients, aged 65 or more, were more likely to have a doctor who worked on his own. There was no such difference in 1977, nor did we find any other difference between the kinds of people using practices with different numbers of doctors.

Comparing their attitudes to various aspects of their general practitioner care, in 1977 those with single-handed doctors or doctors in small partnerships were less likely to feel their doctor had a well-equipped, up-to-date surgery or a pleasant comfortable waiting-room. This can be seen from Table 9.

When asked what they thought were the advantages, if any, from the patient's point of view of a doctor working on his or her own, a

Table 9 Size of partnership and patients' criticisms of surgery and waiting room in 1977

Size of partnership (based on information from patients)	*Proportion of patients who thought their doctor 'not so good' about:*		*Number of patients (= 100%)*
	having a well-equipped up-to-date surgery	*having a pleasant comfortable waiting room*	
Single-handed*	30%	33%	93
Two doctors	23%	36%	139
Three doctors	19%	30%	220
Four doctors	11%	27%	137
Five doctors	7%	21%	42
Six or more	8%	19%	37

* Includes those who thought their doctor probably worked on his or her own.

quarter of those with a single-handed doctor and a half of those with a doctor who worked in a partnership said they did not think there were any. A third of all patients thought one advantage would be that the doctor would know the patient better *personally* and a similar proportion thought that he or she would know the patient better *medically*.

Rather more patients could think of disadvantages than advantages, 72% compared with 56%. The most frequently mentioned disadvantage (by 36%) was that the doctor would be too busy and would not have enough time. This was less often cited as a disadvantage by those with a single-handed doctor, 26% of whom said this compared with 38% of those with a doctor who worked in a partnership. A third of all patients said the single-handed doctor would not always be available, 14% saw an inability for consultation with partners, by either doctor or patients, as a disadvantage, and 10% that there would be longer waiting times in the surgery. In practice, if anything, a slightly *lower* proportion of patients of single-handed doctors said they waited twenty minutes or more the last time they went to the surgery, 30% compared with 41% of those whose doctor worked in a partnership.

There was no evidence of any trends with size of partnership, or of differences between single-handed doctors and others, in patients' views of their doctors in relation to taking his time and not hurrying them; listening to what they say; explaining things to them fully; examining people carefully and thoroughly; keeping people waiting in the waiting room; or always visiting when asked. Neither was there a difference in patients' views on whether their relationship with their doctor was friendly or business-like, but whereas 10% of those with a single-handed doctor wanted their relationship changed (almost always to be more friendly) nearly twice as many, 19%, of those with a doctor who worked with others wanted it changed. Nearly all those who wanted it changed, 97%, wanted it to be more friendly. However, patients with single-handed doctors did not claim to know their doctor any better, nor did they differ in their satisfaction with the care they had received from him or her. They had also been with the same doctor for similar lengths of time. These findings agree with the conclusion in 1964 that people's relationships with and opinions about their doctor vary remarkably little with the number of doctors in the practice.

Partnerships – the doctor's perspective

In the earlier study it was found that while working in partnerships apparently made little difference to their patients, doctors in partnerships said they enjoyed their work more than did doctors working on their own. There was no such difference in this study. Probably most of those who were discontented with single-handed practice had gone into partnership by 1977. There were still a number of differences in the attitudes as well as in the conditions of work between those working single-handed and others, and on a number of issues there were trends with the number of doctors they worked with.

Older doctors of 60 or more were more likely to work on their own, (25% of them did so compared with 11% of younger doctors) and there was a clear fall in the proportion of doctors working on their own or with one partner from 54% of those aged 60 or more to 24% of those under 40. This can be seen from *Table 10.* Put another way, a quarter of single-handed doctors were aged 60 or more compared with a tenth of those in partnerships.

As only 4% of younger doctors (aged under 40) worked on their own it would seem that single-handed practice is likely to disappear fairly rapidly and the views of the doctors would seem to confirm

Table 10 Doctor's age and size of partnership

	Date of birth				*All doctors*
	Before 1917	*1917–1926*	*1927–1936*	*1937 or later*	
	%	%	%	%	%
On own	25	14	12	4	12
With one partner	29	31	20	20	25
With two	16	24	31	29	26
With three	20	22	18	27	22
With four	5	5	8	14	8
With five or more	5	4	11	6	7
Average number of doctors	2.68	2.91	3.33	3.49	3.14
Number of doctors (= 100%)	44	118	120	71	360

this. When asked if they thought partnerships were an advantage or a disadvantage from the viewpoint of the doctor, single-handed doctors were much less likely to perceive them as an advantage, 38% did so compared with 89% of doctors working in partnerships, but of the single-handed more thought partnerships an advantage than a disadvantage. A similar pattern emerged in relation to the advantages or disadvantages to patients. Single-handed doctors were much less likely to regard partnerships as an advantage and more likely than other doctors to see them as a disadvantage, but even so only a minority, a fifth, regarded them as a disadvantage. The figures are in *Table 11*.

Some of the reasons why nine-tenths of the general practitioners who worked in a partnership saw it as an advantage to the doctors are implied by the analyses in *Table 12* (see page 20).

The average number of nights a week doctors said they were on call declined markedly with the number of partners they worked with and there was a general rise in the amount of ancillary help and facilities available with increasing numbers of doctors in the partnership. Single-handed doctors were not only the least likely to have an ECG machine in their practice, they were also comparatively unlikely to have direct access to ECGs. This relative absence of

Table 11 Views of doctors on partnerships as an advantage or disadvantage to patients and general practitioners

	To general practitioners		*To patients*	
	Single-handed doctors	*Doctors in partnerships*	*Single-handed doctors*	*Doctors in partnerships*
Partnerships seen as:	%	%	%	%
Advantage	38	89	24	79
Disadvantage	22	2	21	3
Mixed – equally balanced	33	7	34	14
Uncertain	7	2	21	4
Number of doctors (= 100%)	42	300	42	303

facilities may be why single-handed general practitioners carry out fewer procedures themselves; their average score* was 4.8 compared with 5.7 for doctors in partnerships.

Trainees and medical students were rarely attached to single-handed practices (see *Table 12*) and as a corollary few single-handed doctors were trainers; 7% compared with 18% of doctors in partnership.

With all these differences it is perhaps surprising that being in a partnership or not appeared to be unrelated to their enjoyment of their work. However, it was associated with some of the things they mentioned as contributing to their enjoyment and frustration in their work, although here again the most notable thing is the relative lack of difference. The only statistically significant differences were that single-handed doctors were more likely to say that there was nothing about their work which they found frustrating (16% compared with 3%) but fewer of the single-handed doctors mentioned the variety or unpredictability of their work as something they enjoyed (13% against 26% of doctors in partnership) and fewer of them commented on their freedom or independence (15% compared with 28%). The observed difference in the proportion saying that they found excessive demands of some patients

* For details see Appendix VI.

Table 12 Size of partnerships and various facilities

	Single-handed	*One partner*	*Two partners*	*Three partners*	*Four or more partners*	*All doctors*
Average no. of nights a week on call	3.8	2.9	1.9	1.6	1.4	2.3
Average no. of secretaries or receptionists	2.0	3.2	4.6	5.4	6.5	4.5
Proportion with:						
attached nurse	27%	67%	74%	77%	71%	67%
employed nurse	27%	27%	27%	46%	56%	35%
attached health visitor	74%	89%	85%	90%	96%	88%
attached midwife	70%	80%	77%	85%	90%	80%
an appointment system	73%	82%	92%	96%	94%	88%
treatment room	47%	73%	77%	86%	92%	77%
access to hospital beds	25%	39%	45%	48%	50%	43%
hospital appointment	34%	33%	35%	51%	50%	40%
direct access to ECG	51%	49%	56%	65%	71%	58%
ECG machine in practice	13%	29%	39%	56%	60%	40%
a peak flow meter or vitallo-graph	64%	75%	78%	85%	81%	77%
a refrigerator	87%	93%	92%	96%	100%	94%
Practice has:						
trainees,	2%	15%	24%	44%	44%	26%
medical students on a regular basis	7%	27%	23%	46%	40%	30%
Number of doctors (=100%) *	42	85	92	74	51	351

* When the base relates to more than one set of percentages the minimum has been quoted.

frustrating (33% of single-handed doctors, 41% of those in partnerships) did not reach a level of statistical significance and this ties up with a lack of difference in their estimates of the proportion of consultations that they found trivial, unnecessary, or inappropriate. In spite of the difference in the number of nights they were on call single-handed doctors were no more likely to say they were frustrated by lack of leisure or free time than doctors in partnerships. This was a cause of frustration that we have already shown had declined markedly since 1964.

Evidence that single-handed general practitioners put a rather different emphasis on some aspects of their role than doctors in partnership comes from two questions about the importance of continuity of care and of family care. Doctors were asked: 'In general, how important do you think it is for patients to see the same individual doctor for separate episodes of illness?' and 'How important do you think it is, in general, for different members of a family to go to the same doctor?' Replies are shown in *Table 13*.

With continuity the difference was between single-handed doctors

Table 13 Views on the importance of continuity of care and family care by size of partnership

	Single-handed	*One partner*	*Two partners*	*Three partners*	*Four or more partners*	*All doctors*
	%	%	%	%	%	%
Continuity of care:						
Very important	58	31	26	27	31	33
Fairly „	35	45	50	54	50	47
Relatively unimportant	7	24	24	18	19	20
Other comment	—	—	—	1	—	—
Family care:	%	%	%	%	%	%
Very important	49	32	24	18	13	26
Fairly important	40	46	50	56	46	49
Relatively unimportant	11	22	26	26	39	25
Other comment	—	—	—	—	2	—
Numbers of doctors (=100%)	45	89	95	77	52	363

and those in partnerships, with twice as many proportionally of the former regarding it as very important, 58% against 29%. Over family care too there was a marked difference between single-handed doctors and others but there was also a clear trend with those in larger partnerships regarding it as less important than those in smaller ones.

As single-handed practice becomes less common does this mean that family care and continuity of care are also declining?

Continuity of care

The lengths of time patients aged twenty-one or more had had the same doctor in 1964 and in 1977 are shown in *Table 14*. There was a decline in the proportion who had had the same doctor for 15 years or more but the change was not dramatic given the general increase in mobility. The proportion of people who had changed their address in one year increased from 9.9% of the total population in 1961 to 10.9% in 1971 (OPCS Demographic Review 1977:79).

Table 14 Time with present doctor

	1964	*1977*
	%	%
Less than a year	9	10
One year but less than two years	6	9
Two years but less than five years	17	18
Five years but less than ten years	17	18
Ten years but less than fifteen years	15	15
Fifteen years or more	36	30
Number of patients aged 21 or more (= 100%)	1381	784

Continuity of care is not simply being registered with the same doctor over a long period, it also depends on seeing the same doctor in the practice. Early in the interview patients whose doctor worked with others were asked if they knew the doctor whose list they were on much better than the others, a little better, no better, or less well and if they said no better or less well they were then asked: 'Is there another doctor in the practice whom you really feel you know best and whom you regard as your doctor even though you're not actually registered with him?' If they said there was, then that doctor has been taken as their doctor and all subsequent questions about their doctor related to him or her. The position is summarized in *Table 15.*

Table 15 Patients' identification of doctor within practice

	%
Other doctor in practice regarded as their doctor	11
Knows own doctor:	
much better than the others	49
a little better	19
no better	19
less well	2
Number of patients whose doctor worked with others (=100%)	692

All patients who had consulted a general practitioner in the twelve months before the interview were asked who they had seen mainly during that time. Half had seen their own doctor only, a quarter their own doctor mainly, one in eight had seen partners or a locum as often as their doctor, and one in eight had seen partners or a locum more often than their own doctor. The proportion who had seen their own doctor only declined from 85% of those with doctors in single-handed practices to 49% of those whose doctor worked with one other doctor and down to 40% of those with doctors in larger partnerships of five or more doctors. Four-fifths of patients with a doctor in a partnership reckoned that they could arrange to see their own doctor fairly easily if they wanted to and when asked: 'If you could see another doctor in the group straight away or wait about half an hour and see your own doctor, which would you usually prefer to do?' over half, 55%, said they would wait for their own doctor, about a third, 35%, said they would usually see the other doctor, a tenth that it would depend.

As the ability to seek a second opinion within the practice is sometimes stressed as an advantage of partnerships, patients were asked how easy it was for them to go to another doctor in the same partnership. The majority, 58%, said it was 'very easy', 28% described it as 'fairly easy', 4% as 'rather difficult', and 1% as 'very difficult'; 9% did not know. The proportions describing it as difficult did not vary with the size of the partnership, but patients with doctors in relatively small partnerships of two or three doctors were rather more likely to say it was 'very easy' to see another doctor in the same group or partnership than those with doctors in partnerships of four or more: 63% against 54%.

Finally, all patients were asked how they would feel if they went to the surgery and found unexpectedly that their doctor was not there. Only a small minority, 6%, said they would feel 'quite put out because they could not see their own doctor', a majority, 57%, would feel 'quite prepared to see the other doctor, although they would prefer to see their own doctor', while 34% said they would 'not mind in the least', and 3% made other comments. So the majority of patients feel they can see their own doctor when they want to and while most of them appreciate this aspect of care they do not feel strongly about it, possibly because they tend to take it for granted. It may be acceptable to see a different doctor when you feel you can see your own doctor usually or when you particularly want to do so. Indeed the proportion who said they would not mind about seeing another doctor was higher among those who said they could arrange to see their own doctor fairly easily than among those who could not do so: 36% compared with 25%.

As expected, the length of time patients had had their doctor was related to the age of both the patient and of the doctor. In 1977, with the age of patients, there was not so much a trend as a 'cut-off' point around 45; under that age the estimated average length of time patients had had the same doctor was 7.8 years; for older people it was 10.6 years. There were few differences and no trends within these two broad age groups. There was a clear trend with the doctor's age: 46% of patients whose doctor was 60 or more had been with him or her for at least 15 years and this fell to 23% of patients whose doctor was aged 40–49, to 6% when the doctor was 30–39, and obviously none at all when the doctor was under 30.

Although a relatively high proportion of single-handed doctors were elderly (aged 60 or more), the length of time patients had had their doctor was unrelated to the number of doctors he or she worked with. When the length of time patients had been with the same *practice* is considered a different pattern emerges: partnerships of three or four doctors would seem to be the most stable in the sense that 55% of patients in that size of practice had been in the same practice for fifteen years or more compared with 45% of patients in other practices.

The basic question is how much does continuity of care matter? Some trends are shown in *Table 16*. Some of the differences arose because of variations in the patients' ages. When this was held constant the association between continuity of care and regarding the doctor as easy to talk to no longer reached a level of significance. Among patients aged 45 or more the other associations remained while for the younger patients the length of time they had been with their doctor was not related to their willingness to discuss a personal problem with him or her. For older patients though, it would seem that the longer they had had their doctors the more comfortable and relaxed they felt with them. Continuity of care was *not* related to patients' assessments of whether or not their doctor was good about taking his or her time, not hurrying them or explaining things fully, or listening to what they had to say, or examining people carefully and thoroughly.

So continuity of care would seem to affect the way the patients felt and behaved rather than their assessments of their doctor's behaviour. However, possibly because of a greater sense of identification or loyalty the proportion of patients who said they felt very satisfied with the care they had received from their own doctor increased with the length of time they had been with their doctor.

Given the greater feeling of ease longer-standing patients had with their doctor it is perhaps surprising that they were not even more likely to discuss a personal problem with him or her. The trend from 23% to 33% only just reaches a level of statistical significance. But of course being with the same doctor for a long time is no advantage if you do not have or develop a satisfactory relationship. And for some people it may simply reflect an inability to change their doctor – or a reluctance to go through the procedure that this involves.

Changing and choosing doctors

In the first chapter it was shown that the proportion of patients who

Table 16 Continuity of care and patients' relationships with their doctor

	Length of time had present doctor						*All patients*
	Less than 1 year	*1 year < 2 years*	*2 years < 5 years*	*5 years < 10 years*	*10 years < 15 years*	*15 years or more*	
Might discuss personal problem with own doctor	23%	28%	24%	27%	30%	33%	28%
Knows own doctor 'very well'	5%	13%	4%	16%	23%	32%	18%
Considers doctor to be something of a personal friend	23%	17%	25%	26%	34%	45%	32%
Regards doctor as easy to talk to	76%	78%	74%	80%	82%	87%	80%
'Very satisfied' with own care	34%	36%	47%	44%	53%	59%	49%
Number of patients (=100%)	52	59	140	143	111	215	720

had no choice of doctor in that they reckoned there was no other practice within a reasonable distance* increased from 14% in 1964 to 19% in 1977. There was no evidence of an increase in the number of people changing their doctor and in both studies the most frequent reasons for change were that the patient had moved (47% in 1964, 51% in 1977) or that the doctor had retired, moved, or died (42% in 1964, 39% in 1977).

Ten per cent of the patients in both studies said they had thought of changing their present doctor. In 1977 they were also asked how easy they thought it would be to change to another doctor in a different practice 'just supposing that for some reason you did not get on with your present doctor'. Half thought it would be easy (22% said 'very easy', 28% 'fairly easy'), over a quarter, 28%, thought it would be difficult, and a fifth, 22%, did not know. The main reasons for thinking it would be difficult were that other doctors already had as many patients as they could cope with (30% of those who thought it would be difficult gave this as a reason), that there were few or no other doctors in the area (27% said this), or that there would be a problem explaining why they had left their previous doctor (14%).

The ways in which they had chosen their doctor were similar on the two studies. In 1977 38% had 'inherited' their doctor when he or she took over from another one, 22% chose him or her because he or she was near, 21% said he or she was recommended to them, 10% had had him or her since childhood, and 6% went to their husband's or wife's doctor when they married. Four per cent had met or known him or her before, 3% consulted him or her in an emergency, and 2% said all the other doctors in their area had a full list. One per cent had wanted a woman doctor.**

Although many people 'choose' their doctor in a fairly casual way they rarely changed him or her unless they had to and in 1977 as many as 45% said that either they themselves or their doctor had moved since they first started consulting him or her. Eighty-five per cent of these people said they had not changed their doctor then because they had wanted to keep the same doctor, nearly half of

* 'Is his/her practice the nearest one to you? If 'yes', are there any others reasonably near?'

** The percentages add to more than 100 as a few patients gave more than one way.

them said the surgery was still reasonably near, and one in eight that it was too much trouble to change. (Several gave more than one answer.)

Physical accessibility is obviously an important criterion in selecting a general practitioner and in both 1964 and 1977 about half of the patients said their doctor's practice was the one nearest to them.

Accessibility

Between the two studies there was an increase in the proportion of patients using private transport to get to their general practitioner's surgery from 23% in 1964 to 42% in 1977. This was accompanied by a decline in the proportion who usually walked all the way which fell from 55% to 43%. In spite of these changes the proportion of patients who estimated that they could get to the surgery within five minutes fell from 29% in 1964 to 23% in 1977. This reduction in accessibility seems to be associated with the increase in partnerships. In 1977 the proportion of patients who could get to their doctor's surgery in less than five minutes was a third of those with single-handed doctors compared with a fifth of those whose doctor worked with others.

Sometimes accessibility and continuity may be alternatives for patients and choosing between them will create a conflict. The proportion who had been with the same doctor for fifteen years or longer increased from 23% of those who could get to the surgery in less than five minutes to 44% of those who took half an hour or more to get there.

In terms of being able to get hold of a doctor in an emergency similar proportions of patients in both 1964 and 1977 (one in seven) said they, or their husband or wife, had tried to do this in the previous twelve months.* The length of time before a doctor saw the patient was also similar on the two studies. In 1977 just over half were seen within thirty minutes, another fifth within an hour, while for one in ten the delay was three hours or more. However, the sort of doctor who was seen was rather different and in 1977 more were seen by

* 'During the last twelve months have you (or your husband/wife) tried to get hold of your doctor in a hurry, or in the evening, or at night at all – for yourself, your husband/wife or your children?'

deputizing services, 18% compared with 8% or less in 1964. This increase in deputizing is discussed later in this chapter.

Physical proximity and the immediacy of care in an emergency are two aspects of accessibility but appointment systems and waiting times also contribute to the accessibility of the general practitioner and these are discussed next.

Appointment systems

In 1964 15% of the patients said their doctor had an appointment system. By 1977 this proportion had multiplied by five to 75%. Data from the earlier study showed that waiting times were substantially less when there was an appointment system. In the more recent survey the differences were much less and overall waiting times* had only fallen slightly in spite of the great increase in appointment systems. The figures are in *Table 17.*

Table 17 Waiting times reported by patients

	Appointment system		*No appointment system*		*All patients*	
	1964	*1977*	*1964*	*1977*	*1964*	*1977*
Wait last time:	%	%	%	%	%	%
Less than 10 minutes	49	31	18	16	23	28
10<20	25	35	30	26	29	33
20<30	10	14	19	17	17	15
30<45	10	9	15	18	14	12
45<1 hr	2	5	8	8	7	5
1 hr<1½ hrs	3	4	7	6	7	4
1½ hrs<2 hrs	1	1	2	7	2	2
2 hrs+	—	1	1	3	1	1
Wait reasonable:	%	%	%	%	%	%
Yes	95	87	89	79	90	86
No	5	13	11	21	10	14
Number of patients (= 100%)	179	522	989	151	1196	691

* These were estimated by the patients who were asked: 'The last time you went to the doctor's surgery do you remember how long you had to wait?'

Table 18 Views of waiting times

	Proportion who felt wait unreasonable	
	1964	*1977*
Less than 10 minutes	0% (261)	1% (191)
10< 20	1% (346)	4% (225)
20< 30	2% (207)	12% (101)
30< 45	11% (170)	34% (80)
45<1hr	22% (81)	50% (38)
1hr< 1½ hrs	51% (79)	58% (31)
1½ hrs or longer	69% (32)	52% (25)

The proportion who regarded the time they had to wait as unreasonable had increased on the later study. This appears to be a reflection of changing expectations. *Table 18* shows that on the later study higher proportions of patients regarded waits of between twenty minutes and one hour as unreasonable.

Rather surprisingly there was no indication that people were more likely to regard a wait of the same time as unreasonable if they had an appointment than if they waited in turn.

Sitting in the waiting room may be irritating and frustrating but delays in getting an appointment are potentially a greater barrier to speedy care. Patients were asked how soon they could usually get an appointment when they wanted to see their doctor at the surgery as soon as possible. Almost two-thirds, 63%, said they could usually get an appointment within 24 hours, 15% said it was usually within 48 hours, 8% within three days, and 7% that it was three days or more, (less than 0.5% said it took at least a week). The others were not prepared to generalize. Ritchie and others (1980) report similar results. They found 8% waiting four days or more for an appointment. The estimates from the doctors were less extreme: fewer, 53%, thought it was within 24 hours and more, 34%, that it would be within 48 hours. Only 3% thought it would usually be three days or more before patients could get an appointment. Most of the patients, 84%, thought the time it took was reasonable; the proportion who regarded it as unreasonable rose from 3% of those who said they could usually get an appointment within 24 hours to 33% of those for whom it took between one and three days, and 71% of those who said it took three days or more.

There seemed to be less satisfaction with the way the decision about how soon they should get an appointment was taken. For the great majority, 91%, the decision was made by the secretary or receptionist; 4% said it was made by the doctor, 2% by the patient, and 3% that it was a joint decision. Just over half, 54%, thought this worked very well, 36% that it worked fairly well, but 9% thought it did not work well (1% made other comments). Again this was related to the time it took them to get an appointment, the proportion feeling it worked well dropping from 65% of those who could get one within 24 hours to 17% of those for whom it took three days or more. The proportion who thought it worked well was also higher, 80%, if the doctor was responsible for the decision than if it was a secretary or receptionist, 51%.

Comments suggest some of the things liked and disliked about the arrangement. First from those who thought it worked very well:

> 'The receptionist asks when you want to come and she always tries to fit you in so it's okay.'

> 'I've never had any difficulty, so I imagine it's like the hairdresser's and they take what's free.'

> 'I think it's pretty fair. I think a lot of confusion happens if you don't tell the receptionist it's urgent. A lot of people say they can't get an appointment today, but they don't explain it properly.'

Then from those who thought the arrangement worked 'fairly well':

> 'They don't ask you any questions. She just gives you the earliest date, irrespective of why you want to see the doctor'.

> 'She does ask you what you want to see him for – and if it's something urgent she will try and fit you in – she's good like that.'

> 'This one up here – she can be awkward with some and won't get them in, but she's been alright with me because I've not taken "no" for an answer from her. She's refused my wife the same day though. I don't really like it. I don't like one receptionist picking some and not picking others. She doesn't ask what time you'd like, she just chooses the time.'

And from those who thought it did not work well:

> 'You don't know if she's under instruction not to take too many or

what, but you always have the feeling she'd rather you didn't come. It's just her attitude when you speak to her.'

'It's not right. Why should they pick and choose, they're not there to look after you, they're only there to put your name down at the nearest time. They want pensioning off in my opinion. I've been there and seen them put my name down for two days later and I could see on the sheet that she had free appointments earlier than that. What can you do? If you moan, you're up the road again – you get nowt. If your face doesn't fit with them two, you're out'.

One in eight of the patients whose doctor had an appointment system said that they had put off going to see their doctor on some occasion in the last twelve months because of the need for an appointment. This proportion rose from 8% of those who said they could usually get an appointment within 24 hours to 40% of those who said they usually had to wait for three days or more. So delays in getting appointments certainly seem to act as barriers to general practitioner care.

But if some doctors attempt to use such barriers in order to reduce their 'trivial' consultations they appear to be unsuccessful. The average proportion of surgery consultations estimated by the doctors as being trivial, inappropriate, or unnecessary was 31% if patients said they could usually get an appointment within three days, and higher, 44%, if it took longer. It may be that doctors who feel alienated from their patients put up such barriers. The extent of the delay was not related to the size of partnership although, as will be shown in a later chapter, it tended to be longer for doctors who worked at a health centre.

A summary view of patients' attitudes to and experiences of appointment systems is given by their preference for continuing with their present arrangement (waiting in turn or an appointment system) or changing to the other type of arrangement. Nineteen per cent of those whose doctor had an appointment system said they would prefer to 'wait in turn' while 25% of those who waited in turn would prefer an appointment system. So in both situations the majority would prefer to keep the current arrangement and the proportions opting for change did not differ significantly.

Amongst those whose doctor had an appointment system preference for one was related to the length of time it took to get an appointment (declining from 86% of those who could usually get one within 24 hours to 49% of those who said it usually took three days or more), the length of time they had to wait at the surgery (declining from 91% who had waited less than ten minutes to 42% of those who waited an hour or more), and to how they made an appointment (it was 83% of those who phoned from home, 63% if they depended on neighbours or had to go round to the surgery to get an appointment). This last difference was related to social class variations in attitudes to appointment systems as working class patients were less able to phone from their own home or from work,

Table 19 Social class and appointments

	Middle class	*Working class*	*All patients*
	%	%	%
How usually makes an appointment:			
Phones from home	72	45	56
Phones from work	13	4	8
Uses a neighbour's phone	3	7	5
Goes to a public telephone	4	23	16
Goes to the surgery	6	17	12
Other	2	4	3
Number of patients (= 100%)	198	272	490
	%	%	%
Preference of those with appointment system:			
Likes it	89	70	79
Would prefer to wait in turn	9	28	19
Other	2	2	2
Number of patients (= 100%)	261	342	625
	%	%	%
Preference of those without appointment system:			
Would like appointment system	29	22	25
Rather wait in turn as now	71	75	73
Other	—	3	2
Number of patients (= 100%)	65	99	170

and more of them would prefer to change from an appointment system to waiting in turn.* This is shown in *Table 19*.

Doctors' views of appointment systems are summarized in their opinions about whether appointment systems were an advantage or a disadvantage for patients and for doctors. Overall a higher proportion thought it an advantage for doctors, 80%, than for patients, 65%. Perceptions on both scores were clearly related to whether they had an appointment system or not (see *Table 20*).

Table 20 Doctors' views on appointment systems

	Doctor has appointment system for:			
	All surgery consultations	*Some surgery consultations*	*No surgery consultations*	*All doctors*
For doctors:	%	%	%	%
An advantage	89	63	52	80
A disadvantage	2	14	22	7
Mixed – equally balanced	9	23	26	13
For patients:	%	%	%	%
An advantage	80	44	15	65
A disadvantage	2	31	53	14
Mixed – equally balanced	18	25	32	21
Number of doctors (= 100%)	248	71	41	362

A final point on accessibility is that doctors who were accessible in one way were more likely to be accessible in another. If patients could get an appointment within 24 hours they waited less long in the surgery than those who had a delay in getting an appointment. This can be seen from *Table 21*.

* For a description of social class classifications see Appendix V.

Table 21 Time to get an appointment and time kept waiting at the surgery

	Time to get an appointment			
	Less than 24 hrs	*Within 48 hrs*	*Within 3 days*	*3 days or longer*
Wait last time:	%	%	%	%
Less than 10 mins	35	23	20	15
10 minutes < 20	38	31	28	40
20 minutes < 30	12	17	18	18
30 minutes < 45	7	13	18	12
45 minutes < 1 hr	3	10	5	6
1 hour < 1½ hours	4	4	8	—
1½ hours or more	1	2	3	9
Number of patients (= 100%)	330	78	39	33

Family care

Earlier in this chapter we showed that half the doctors regarded family care as 'fairly important', a quarter as 'very important', and the other quarter as 'relatively unimportant'. The importance doctors attached to family care was greatest for those who worked in single-handed practice and declined with increasing size of partnership. Does this imply that family care is becoming less common? Which patients receive family care and which doctors give it? How much difference does family care make to patient–doctor relationships and the care that patients receive?

One criterion of whether or not a patient has a family doctor is whether he or she has the same doctor as other relatives living in the same household. The proportion of people living with relatives who all had the same doctor was 72% in 1964 and a similar proportion, 74%, in 1977. But whereas 23% in the earlier study had entirely different doctors, this proportion had fallen to 15% in the more recent one while the proportion with a different doctor in the same partnership had risen from 5% to 11%. The proportion of patients who had the same doctor as other relatives who did not live with them increased from 39% to 45%. So, on this mechanistic definition there was no evidence that family doctoring had declined. The difficult problem then and now is to pinpoint the implications. As might be expected those who had the same doctor or partnership as other relatives in the same household were more likely to have had a home visit by one of the doctors to some member of their household: 82% compared with 62% of people living with relatives who had quite different doctors. But we have not found any differences in patients' attitudes, relating to whether or not they had a family doctor.

For the doctors, it is difficult to determine either the extent to which they practise family medicine or the effect of practising it. A recent editorial in the Journal of the Royal College of General Practitioners (1979) maintained:

> 'Although family doctors know instinctively from their day-to-day practice that looking after several members of the family is of fundamental importance and offers unique and valuable insights into the care of individual members of those families, family medicine as a discipline has largely failed to provide satisfactory scientific evidence to convince colleagues in other branches of medicine.'

Night calls and deputizing services

With the increase in partnerships it might be expected that individual doctors would not be on call for so many nights a week and that the need for an outside deputizing service to attend emergencies and night calls would have declined. The first expectation was borne out but not the second.

The proportion of doctors on call for five or more nights a week had fallen from 39% in 1964 to 9% in 1977. This could not be explained just by a decrease in the proportion of single-handed doctors as for them the proportion on call for five or more nights a week had also fallen, from 72% to 42%. This last proportion declined to 12% for those with one partner, 3% for those with two and none of those in larger partnerships.

In 1964, 9% of the general practitioners said they sometimes used an 'emergency call' service. By 1977 26% said they used a deputizing service regularly and another 18% used one occasionally. The proportion using one at all fell from 56% of those in single-handed practices to 31% of those in partnerships of five or more doctors. Twenty-nine per cent of those who used one regularly said they personally were not usually on call on any night of the week, compared with 3% of those who used one occasionally and 1% of those who never used one. Older doctors, of 60 or more, were more likely to use a deputizing service, three-fifths of them used one regularly or occasionally compared with two-fifths of the younger doctors. Members of the Royal College of General Practitioners in contrast were less likely to use a deputizing service, a third of them used one regularly or occasionally, compared with almost half the other doctors. In general it seemed that those using deputizing services were less enamoured of their work than other doctors. They regarded a higher proportion of their consultations as trivial, inappropriate, or unnecessary, were less likely to say they enjoyed their work as a general practitioner 'very much' and carried out fewer procedures. This can be seen from *Table 22.*

Table 22 Views and practices of doctors using deputizing services

	Doctors using deputizing service:	
	Regularly or occasionally	*Never*
Average proportion of consultations felt to be trivial, inappropriate, or unnecessary	38%	28%
Enjoys general practice 'very much'	49%	61%
Average procedure score*	5.1	6.1
Number of doctors (=100%)	155	199

* For details see Appendix VI.

Nearly all the doctors who used a deputizing service at all, 95%, saw it as an advantage for the doctor, but only 62% of those who did not use one thought this. Just over half of all the doctors, 52%, saw it as a disadvantage for the patient and this proportion was 79% of those who did not use one, 23% of those who used it occasionally, and 16% of those who used it regularly.

On both studies patients were asked what arrangements their doctor had for night calls, and similar proportions, just over half on each study, did not know. On the more recent study 14% (or 31% of those who had any idea what the arrangements were) thought he or she used a deputizing or emergency doctor service. Patients were also asked whether they preferred their doctor to use a deputizing service or to have some other arrangement. Answers were similar on the two studies with just under a fifth opting for a deputizing service. So the increase in the service had not been accompanied by an increase in its acceptability although preference for a deputizing service was relatively high among those who said their doctor had such an arrangement – but even for them it was still only a minority view. This can be seen from *Table 23* which also shows that a rota between partners was more popular than an arrangement with neighbouring doctors. Among the small group of twenty-two patients with experience of a deputizing service for themselves or their families in the previous twelve months 18% said they preferred such an arrangement – a similar proportion as for all patients, and a further indication that experience of the service did not increase its acceptability. Dixon and Williams (1977) in their study of 100,000 patient contacts with deputizing services found 'no substantiated evidence of shortcomings in the care' but they made no attempt to assess patients' acceptance of or satisfaction with the service.

Table 23 Patients' preference for deputizing service or other arrangement for night calls in 1977

	Present arrangement for night calls thought to be:					*All patients*
	*Rota with partners**	*Rota with neighbouring doctors**	*Deputizing service*	*Other arrangement**	*Unknown*	
Prefers or would prefer:	%	%	%	%	%	%
Deputizing service	8	17	33	19	18	18
Other arrangement	81	48	47	71	60	63
Don't mind or other comment	11	35	20	10	22	19
*Number of patients (=100%)***	192	52	112	31	449	814

*Patients with these arrangements were asked if they would prefer a deputizing service or their present arrangement.

** A few patients mentioned more than one arrangement.

Equipment

Finally, in our review of the changes in the setting in which general practice is carried out we should consider the equipment which was available. Here our comparisons are with a survey of 157 general practitioners who were interviewed in 1963 (Cartwright and Marshall 1965).

As can be seen from *Table 24* the proportion of general practitioners who had a refrigerator at their practice had risen between 1963 and 1977 but the proportion with a haemoglobinometer and with a microscope had fallen. These last two changes may be related to differences in access to various diagnostic procedures in hospital which are discussed later, in Chapter 6. A survey of 576 general practitioners in 1969 (Irvine and Jefferys 1971) reported that 68% of the doctors had vaginal specula and 10% an electrocardiograph. So the availability of these had increased appreciably.

Table 24 Equipment

	Proportion of doctors with this equipment at practice in		*Proportion of those who did not have this equipment in 1977 who wanted it*
	1963	*1977*	
Refrigerator	82%	94%	32% (22)
Microscope	52%	46%	18% (188)
Haemoglobinometer	48%	36%	14% (228)
Vaginal specula	*	99%	** (4)
ECG machine	*	40%	53% (211)
A vision testing chart	*	98%	** (8)
Peak flow meter or vitallograph	*	77%	18% (80)
Number of doctors (=100%)	155	365	

* Not asked in 1963.
** Base numbers too small.

When the patients described their doctors as good about having a well-equipped, up-to-date surgery, they were in fact better equipped than doctors who were regarded as 'not so good'. For example when patients described a doctor as good about having a well-equipped surgery 42% of doctors had an ECG machine but this proportion fell to 24% among doctors described as 'not so good' about this. Corresponding figures for a refrigerator were 95% of the well-equipped doctors, 88% of the not so well equipped, and for a peak flow meter or vitallograph 81% and 62% for the two groups.

Summing up

The decline in single-handed practice and the increase in partnerships with three or more doctors appears to have had little effect on the nature of general practitioner care or on patient-doctor relationships. The extent of family care and of continuity of care had changed remarkably little in the thirteen years between the two studies. There were some changes in accessibility and in the more recent study patients took longer to reach their doctor but waited a slightly shorter time in the waiting room. The reduction in waiting times was less than might have been expected from the great increase in appointment systems, and these may have benefitted the doctor more than the patients. Although most patients reckoned they could get an appointment within 24 hours when they wanted to see their doctor as soon as possible, the fact that 15% thought it would take more than two days is probably a cause for some concern, as is the marked increase in the use of deputizing services.

The main picture from the data in this chapter is of quite major changes in the organisation of the general practitioner service alongside small and mainly insignificant changes in the basic relationship between patients and doctors.

3 Changes in the frequency and nature of doctor-patient contacts

How, if at all, has the frequency with which patients contact their general practitioners changed? And have there been any changes in the place or the nature of these consultations and how patients and doctors feel about them? These are the questions tackled in this chapter which starts by looking at an area in which there has been a marked change: home visits.

Home visits

The amount of home visiting done by general practitioners declined substantially between 1964 and 1977. This is shown by the number of home visits reported by patients in the last twelve months (see *Table 25*) and by the proportion of consultations during the two

Table 25 Home visits to patients

No. of home visits during previous twelve months	*1964*	*1977*
	%	%
None	77	81
One	8	10
Two – four	8	6
Five – nine	3	2
Ten or more	4	1
Number of patients (= 100%)	1394	834

weeks before the interview which took place in the home: this fell from 22% to 13%.

Data from the General Household Survey which covers all ages also shows a decline in the proportion of home visits from 22% in the first, 1971, study to 16% in 1977.* Nevertheless, in comparison with North America, doctors in this country still visit people's homes relatively frequently. In the United States the proportion of home visits declined from 9.7% to 2.3% (US Department of Health, Education and Welfare 1971) in the ten years 1959 to 1969 and the place of consultation is not recorded in more recent publications.

Some doctors (Stevenson 1976 and Williams 1970) have associated the fall in home visits with an increase in appointment systems but there was no association between the two in the 1977 study and in 1964 a relatively high proportion of patients whose doctor had an appointment system reported a home visit, 28% compared with 22% of those whose doctor did not have one.

One obvious reason for the decline in home visiting here is the increase in private transport. In the last chapter we showed that the proportion of patients who normally travelled to their doctor by private transport had increased from 23% in 1964 to 42% in 1977. In 1977 only 12% of people normally using private transport to get to the surgery reported a home visit in the previous twelve months compared with 22% of those who walked or went by public transport. (The difference persisted when age was held constant.) But the increase in the use of private transport by patients did not account for all the fall in home visiting. Among those using private transport the proportion reporting a home visit fell from 19% in 1964 to 12% in 1977.

If private transport makes it quicker for patients to get to the surgery (11% of them travelling in that way took 15 minutes or more to get there compared with 18% of patients who walked all the way and 56% of those using public transport) the increase in the number of cars on the road has added to the time it takes doctors to reach their patients' homes and increased their parking problems. So home visiting has become less attractive to doctors and the increasing facilities available at their surgeries may also make them regard home visits as less appropriate. How much does it matter?

One implication is that as the proportion of patients reporting any home visits in the previous year had fallen general practitioners are

* These figures relate to Great Britain.

likely to be less familiar with their patients' homes. But as members of a family usually have the same doctor a patient's home is visited more often than he or she has a consultation there. A third, 32%, of the adults in 1977 said their general practitioner or his or her partners had visited their home in the last year.* Thirty per cent said it was between one and five years ago, 15% that it was five years or more. Nearly a quarter, 23%, said he or she had never been. This last proportion fell from 42% of those who had been with the same doctor for less than a year to 13% of those who had been with their doctor for ten years or more.

But it was not only the proportion of patients who reported a home visit that fell. Among those who were visited the proportion who had received five or more visits during the year dropped from 29% in 1964 to 19% in 1977. This suggests that the chronically ill may be receiving less attention from their general practitioners.

Young children and old people are of course the most likely to have home visits. The distribution is shown in *Figure 1*. Even so, half

Figure 1 *Variations in the proportion with a name visit for themselves in the previous twelve months by age*

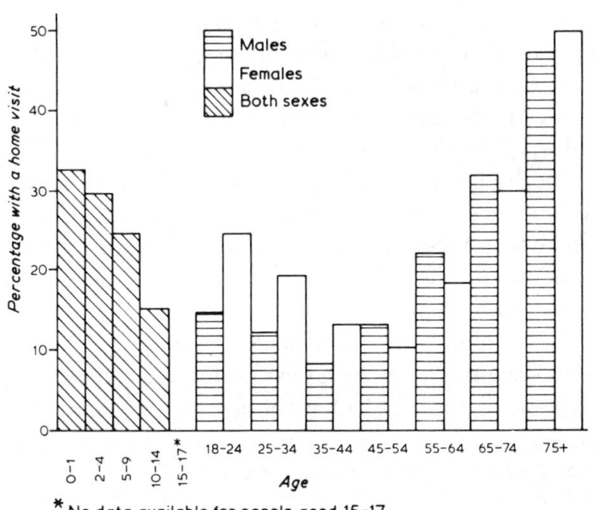

* 'When was the last, most recent time your general practitioner or his partners, etc., came to your home here, professionally, to see you or any other member of your household?'

of those aged 75 or more said they had not had any visits from a general practitioner in the last twelve months. As so many old people now live alone (43% of those aged 75 or more in our sample did so in 1977 compared with 10% of younger people) they do not benefit from doctors' visits to other members of their household. Eleven per cent of those aged 75 or more said their doctor had never visited their home.

The number of home visits patients had received in the last year was clearly related to their satisfaction with their care, to their views of their relationship with their doctor as being friendly rather than businesslike,* to their assessment of whether or not they would consult their doctor about a personal problem that worried them,** and to whether they found their doctor an easy person to talk to.***

The trends remain in the same direction but do not always reach the level of statistical significance when age or social class are held constant. The figures are in *Table 26*, but the interpretation is difficult. Patients who feel at ease with their doctor may be more inclined to ask for a home visit, while patients who have been rebuffed when they have asked for one may feel unhappy about other aspects of their relationship.

The trends in *Table 26* were more pronounced than trends with simply the number of consultations in the previous twelve months. The proportion very satisfied with their care rose from 48% of those with no consultations to 59% of those with ten or more; the proportion who regarded their general practitioner as something of a personal friend from 26% to 43%, and the proportion who thought they might discuss a personal problem with their doctor from 21% to 38%, but there was no trend with the proportion who said they found their doctor easy to talk to. The trends are also similar to, but stronger than, those found with the length of time they had had their doctor (see *Table 16*, page 26).

Gray (1978) maintains: 'Good general practice will always consist of patients feeling at home with their doctor and of doctors feeling at home with their patients.' Our findings suggest that this type of

* 'Do you consider your doctor to be something of a personal friend or is your relationship pretty much a businesslike one?'

** 'If you were worried about a personal problem that *wasn't* a strictly medical one, do you think you might discuss it with *your* doctor?'

*** 'And would you say it is easy to talk to your doctor and ask him questions or do you feel it is not possible to talk to him as much as you'd like?'

Table 26 Home visits and attitudes to their general practitioner

	Number of home visits in previous twelve months				*All patients*
	None	*One*	*Two – Four*	*Five or more*	
Proportion:					
Very satisfied with own care	47%	49%	66%	70%	49%
Considers doctor to be something of a personal friend	28%	41%	45%	55%	32%
Might discuss personal problem with doctor	26%	34%	40%	47%	28%
Regards doctor as easy to talk to	79%	85%	85%	93%	80%
Number of patients (= 100%)	570	79	47	29	726

relationship may be more likely to develop when doctors have seen their patients in their homes. Certainly the decline in home visiting has been accompanied by a fall in the proportion who regarded their doctor as something of a personal friend; 44% in 1964, 32% in 1977.

For the doctors too the decline in home visiting may have its disadvantages, as doctors who enjoy their work are more likely to visit their patients. The proportion of patients reporting a home visit was 20% if their doctors said they enjoyed their work very much or moderately, 10% if they said they did not enjoy it very much or not at all.

What of the future? Are home visits going to continue to decline and almost disappear as in North America? For those of us who hope this will not happen one encouraging sign is that patients with younger doctors were more likely to report a home visit in the last twelve months than patients with older doctors. The proportion rose from 13% of those with doctors aged 60 or more to 19% of those aged 40–59, and to 28% of those with doctors under 40.* (There was no clear association between the ages of doctors and patients.)

This trend in home visits with age is in the opposite direction from that observed on earlier studies (Eimerl and Pearson, 1966; Williams, 1970) and it may be unwise to attach too much weight to it. Other evidence suggests that the decline in home visits may continue. When doctors were asked about the future development of health care and whether they would like to see more or less emphasis on home visiting in general practice just over half, 52%, of the doctors would like to see less emphasis, only 6% wanted more emphasis, and 42% wanted no change.

Whether or not a doctor worked in a health centre, or had a group practice allowance, or was a member of the Royal College of General Practitioners or a trainer were all unrelated to the proportion of patients reporting a home visit. So too were the number of doctors he or she worked with, the number of patients the doctor looked after and the country in which he or she qualified.

Most general practitioners realized that their home visiting had declined. Three-quarters of them thought the proportion of their home visits to surgery consultations had gone down in the last ten years,** just under a fifth that it had not changed, leaving less than one in ten who said it had gone up. While there was general agreement on the recent direction of change in home visiting, there was less unanimity about changes in consultation rates which are considered next.

Consultation rates

Are general practitioner consultation rates rising or falling? Figures from the National Morbidity Survey in 1970–71, based on data from fifty-three practices, found a national average consultation rate of 3.0 compared with one of 3.8 in the earlier 1955–56 study (Royal College of General Practitioners 1974a; Logan and Cushion 1958). From these figures and from those in a number of individual

* The doctor's date of birth was obtained from the Department of Health and Social Security.

** Those who had been in practice between two and ten years were asked about changes during this time.

practices it has been concluded that rates are falling (Howie 1977). On the other hand, data quoted in the 1977 Review Body Report suggested consultation rates had risen by nearly 3% between 1970 and 1975 (Review Body on Doctors' and Dentists' Remuneration 1977).

Data from the General Household Survey cover the period 1971–77, and show a small fall in consultation rates for adults. Their rates are considerably higher than those in the National Morbidity Survey. The probable reason for the difference, discussed in the General Household Survey, 1972, is the non-representative nature of the National Morbidity Survey.

The distribution of the number of consultations patients said they had had during the previous 12 months in our 1977 study is similar to that found on another 1977 survey (Ritchie, Jacoby, and Bone 1980). It terms of changes over time the data from our two studies are equivocal. Comparisons in *Table 27* show a decline in the proportion who had not consulted at all, suggesting an increase in consultation rates. This may have been accompanied by a small decrease in the consultation rate per person consulting, from 5.1 to 4.8. But estimating consultation rates from the data in *Table 27* is a dubious exercise. If midpoints are taken for the 2–4 and 5–9 groups and 12 for the ten or more, then there is no significant change in the overall consultation rate: 3.4 in 1964, 3.6 in 1977. Estimates of annual consultation rates based on the number of reported

Table 27 Patients' estimates of number of general practitioner consultations in previous twelve months*

	1964	*1977*
	%	%
None	34	25
One	15	18
Two – four	26	30
Five – nine	11	14
Ten or more	14	13
No. of patients (= 100%)	1394	825

* 'Now just during the last 12 months, that is since this time last year, how many times have you yourself consulted, that is seen professionally, your doctor – or his partners, assistant, or locum?' **If had doctor less than a year** 'Please include any consultations with your previous general practitioner'.

consultations in the previous two weeks also show a small difference, but in the opposite direction: 4.5 in 1964, 4.3 in 1977.

Most general practitioners in our study, 60%, thought that the average consultation rate per patient on their list had risen in the last ten years, 9% thought it had gone down, 31% that it had not changed.

On balance the direction of the change seems doubtful, and the size of the change is almost certainly small. One possibility is that the proportion of patients consulting has risen but the consultation rate per person consulting has gone down. Is there any evidence of changes in patients' expectations or attitudes which may have influenced either the frequency with which they consult their doctor or the content and nature of the consultation?

Patients' attitudes, expectations, and knowledge

One obvious change is the increase in women using oral contraceptives and in 1975 just over half the current users of professional family planning services went to their general practitioner for this type of help (Bone 1978). When patients aged 25 or more were asked whether there were certain sorts of problems they felt they would be *more* inclined to consult their general practitioner about than they would have been ten years ago, 25% of them said yes compared with only 5% who mentioned things they might be less inclined to consult about. Five per cent of people said they would be more likely to consult about such problems as sex or contraception, 4% mentioned marital or social problems and 2% psychiatric or emotional problems.

In an earlier chapter we saw that most general practitioners thought their patients were now more knowledgeable about health matters and just over half the patients over 25 thought their own knowledge of health matters was greater in 1977. Most of those who felt this thought it was because they had had more experience or were older now but 16% of all patients thought their knowledge was greater because of television, radio, or reading.

> 'I think there's more publications, more talk, more articles, television and discussion.'

If patients are more knowledgeable about their health this may change their hopes and expectations about a consultation with their doctor. Patients who had consulted a doctor in the two weeks before the interview were asked: 'Before you consulted the GP that time what did you think or hope he might do for you? Anything else?' There was a fall in the proportion who said they had hoped for or expected a prescription or some medicine from 52% to 41%. So there seems to be less demand for medication from patients on the later study. The proportion of consultations at which a prescription was given had not changed significantly – in 1977 it was two-thirds. On both studies it was higher than the proportion at which it was expected.

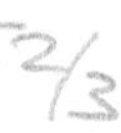

Further evidence that patients' attitudes to drugs had changed comes from the nature of their criticisms about their doctors' prescribing habits. These are shown in *Table 28*. Whereas in 1964 twice as many patients were critical of their doctor for not giving prescriptions as thought he was too inclined to give them, by 1977 the position was reversed. Similar proportions on the two studies, 4%, thought their doctor rather reluctant to give prescriptions but the proportion who thought he was too inclined to do this had trebled. Even so, the great majority of patients, nine-tenths, felt their doctor was reasonable about this. But when asked for their view on doctors in general almost half, 46%, of the patients in 1977 who answered thought doctors were too inclined to give prescriptions while 2% thought they were rather reluctant.

Table 28 Views on doctors' prescribing habits

	1964	*1977*
Felt their doctor was:	%	%
Too inclined to give a prescription	2	7
Rather reluctant to give a prescription	4	4
Reasonable about this	94	89
Number of patients answering question (= 100%)	1159	709

Further data suggesting that the doctors' habit of giving a prescription may lead patients to expect one came from an analysis of patients' expectations by the length of time they had had their doctor. In 1977 only 27% of those who had had their doctor for less than two years said they had expected or hoped for a prescription compared with 47% of those who had had the same doctor for a longer time – a difference falling just short of statistical significance at the 5% level. The position was reversed for expectations about advice or reassurance: 46% against 21%. There were no age variations in either of these, nor were there any significant differences with the length of time they had had their doctor in what happened at the consultation.

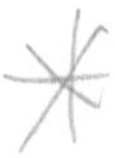

The patient as well as the doctor may contribute to the decision to prescribe, and to some extent the situation in which a prescription is given at most consultations tends to be self-perpetuating. The doctor's training and orientation prompts him or her to take some positive action – so he or she prescribes a drug, then patients come to expect a prescription and doctors perceive themselves as being under pressure to prescribe. But while doctors are likely to be aware of any pressure from patients to prescribe a drug they may be unaware when patients feel doctors turn to their prescription pad

Table 29 Patients' views of doctors who are too inclined to give prescriptions and those who are reasonable or reluctant about this

	Patient regards own doctor as:	
	Too inclined to give prescription	*Reluctant or reasonable about giving prescription*
Would have liked more information about last problem for which consulted doctor	34%	19%
Some occasion in last twelve months when felt doctor might have done more thorough exam*	33%	10%
Would like 10 minutes uninterrupted conversation with a sympathetic doctor	38%	21%
Number of patients (=100%)	36	547

* Those who had not consulted in the last twelve months have been excluded.

too readily. A preference for action is more easily expressed than a preference for inaction.

Patients who felt their doctor was too inclined to write a prescription may have felt they were given a prescription rather than an examination, or information or discussion. This is suggested by the analyses in *Table 29*.

In another study of general practitioner consultations, it was found that fewer medicines were prescribed when the doctor found the patient easy to talk to than when he or she did not (Cartwright 1974).

While patients in 1977 seemed to be less inclined to expect a prescription than they had been in 1964 they more often expressed a desire for advice or reassurance. The proportion expecting or hoping for this before a consultation rose from 18% in 1964 to 29% in 1977 and the proportion who reported that they had been given advice or reassurance at a consultation also rose from 41% to 65%.

This evidence from the patients suggests that in 1977 they were attaching more importance to discussion and rather less to medication than they had done in 1964. Does this mean that they were putting more emphasis on the doctor's social role than they had done at the time of the earlier study? Data about this are examined next.

Consultations for family, social, and psychological problems

In fact the proportion of patients who thought 'a general practitioner was a suitable person to talk to about problems such as children getting into trouble or difficulties between husband and wife' had declined from 40% in 1964 to 30% in 1977. But the proportion who thought they might discuss a personal problem that was not strictly medical with their own doctor if they were worried about it was 28% on both studies. So while people are apparently less likely to regard general practitioners as appropriate for dealing with family or relationship problems, the proportion who reckon they would turn to their general practitioner with a personal problem had not changed. And there was no evidence from our data about consultations in the two weeks before the interview of any increase in consultation for such reasons. The proportion of patients who thought they would consult their general practitioner about a constant feeling of depression for three weeks had, however, increased: it was 54% in 1964, 69% in 1977.

Ninety-two per cent of the general practitioners in our sample in 1977 thought there was a growing tendency for people to seek help from doctors for problems in their family lives. At the same time the proportion of doctors who felt it was appropriate for people to seek help from their general practitioners for such problems had fallen from 87% in 1964 to 67% in 1977.* It would seem that general practitioners' tolerance for such consultations had declined. They may have conveyed some of their feeling about this to patients since by 1977 fewer of them felt it was appropriate to consult about such things.

Another possibility is that the setting up of social services departments may have given both patients and doctors the idea that social workers would be available for this aspect of care. Patients' and doctors' views on the appropriateness of consultation over family problems were related. In 1977 the proportion of patients who did not think a general practitioner a suitable person to talk to about children getting into trouble, or difficulties between husband and wife, was 48% among those whose general practitioner felt it was appropriate to discuss family problems and rose to 62% when the general practitioner regarded it as inappropriate. But there were no differences between the two groups in the proportion who thought they might discuss a personal problem with their doctor, nor in the proportion who regarded him as easy to talk to. Doctors seem to have been unsuccessful in actually discouraging such consultations possibly because of the inadequacy of alternative sources of help over such problems.

The few doctors who did not think that people were more likely to turn to doctors for help over family problems were more likely to regard such consultations as appropriate: 81% of them did so, 66% of other doctors.

The doctors' views were also clearly related to their statements

* The question was slightly different on the two studies. In 1964 we asked 'When patients ask you about such things as children getting into trouble or family discord do you feel it is appropriate for you to be consulted about such things or that such problems are more appropriately discussed with other people?' In 1977 the question was: 'Given present conditions in general practice, do you think it is appropriate for people to seek help from general practitioners for problems in their family lives?'

about their enjoyment of general practice. The proportion who thought it appropriate for general practitioners to be consulted about family problems fell from 77% of those who enjoyed general practice 'very much' to 59% of those who enjoyed it moderately, and to 38% who said they did not enjoy it very much or not at all. However, in terms of cause and effect it is probably more relevant to think of this the other way round: 64% of those who felt it was appropriate said they enjoyed their work very much compared with 39% of those who regarded it as inappropriate. Doctors who used a deputizing service were less likely than others to regard it as appropriate for patients to consult them about family problems: 61% compared with 73% did so.

Among patients, not surprisingly, the proportion who thought they might discuss a personal problem with their doctor was higher, 53%, if they regarded a general practitioner as a suitable person to consult about family problems, than if they were uncertain about this (31% might consult), or if they did not regard a general practitioner as a suitable person (14% might consult). So 7% of all patients predicted that they would consult their own doctor about a personal problem although they did not regard a general practitioner as a suitable person to consult about family problems while 11% said they would not consult their doctor even though they regarded general practitioners in general as suitable. The latter response was clearly related to social class, falling from 26% in Social Class I (Professional) to 3% in Social Class V (Unskilled). Middle-class patients tend to regard general practitioners as appropriate for other people to consult about their personal problems: they themselves generally have alternative sources of support and help. And there may be class variations in the way people perceive such problems.

Frequency of consultation was related both to regarding a doctor as a suitable person to talk to about personal problems and to predictions about whether the patients would consult about a personal problem. The former rose from 21% of those who had not consulted their doctor at all in the previous 12 months to 38% of those who had consulted ten or more times and the latter from 23% to 44%. Familiarity may be the key issue here. Statements about how well they knew their doctor are related to both of these questions and to whether they would consult their doctor about depression. This is shown in *Table 30.* The length of time they had had their doctor did not show such marked trends.

Table 30 Knowledge of and attitudes towards general practitioners

	Patients who know their own doctor:				*Never consulted him*
	Very well	*Reasonably well*	*Fairly well*	*Not very well*	
Regards a general practitioner as a suitable person to talk to about family problems	36%	35%	29%	17%	35%
Might discuss personal problem with their general practitioner	50%	30%	22%	14%	26%
Would consult their general practitioner about depression	72%	75%	69%	58%	67%
Number of patients (= 100%)	148	257	213	155	43

Those who had never consulted their general practitioner tended to fall between those who knew their doctor very well or reasonably well and those who knew him or her fairly well or not very well. This may be because those who feel they know their doctor only fairly well or not very well have had a somewhat negative experience.

An alternative explanation for the associations in *Table 30* is that those who do not regard him or her as an appropriate person to talk to about social or emotional problems do not consult their doctor very often and therefore know him or her less well.

As general practitioners were less likely in 1977 to feel that it was reasonable for patients to consult them about personal problems, and they also felt it was more likely that patients would do so, this might suggest that in 1977 doctors would think a higher proportion of their consultations were for inappropriate reasons. However this does not seem to be the case.

Trivialities

As we showed earlier, in Chapter 1, the proportion of surgery consultations that general practitioners felt were trivial, unnecessary, or inappropriate had not changed between 1964 and 1977.

In the more recent study those doctors who felt it was appropriate to be consulted about family problems thought a smaller proportion of their consultations were trivial, inappropriate, or unnecessary than those doctors who did not feel it was appropriate. The average proportions were 30% and 40% respectively.

When asked for an example of what they considered a trivial, unnecessary, or inappropriate reason for which they had been consulted in the last two weeks, family or personal problems were the fourth most frequently cited illustration. Two-fifths mentioned specific physical conditions which they thought fell into this category: toothache, constipation, colds, sore throats, non-infected insect bite, small scratch, bruised fingers, headaches. A fifth reported conditions which were presented at an inappropriate time – too soon, or after they had cleared up, or as an emergency:

> 'A sore throat of six hours duration.'

> 'Child with a three week history of mild catarrh whose parents demanded immediate attention, interrupting planned surgery.'

> 'Common cold on the first or second day.'

A quarter mentioned unnecessary or inappropriate certificates or form-filling:

> 'Recovered from influenza but needing a certificate.'

> 'The person who just needs a certificate to show an employer for one or two days off work.'

Ten per cent mentioned family or personal problems which they classified in this way:

> 'Matrimonial problems concerning divorce proceedings which more appropriately belong to the legal profession.'

> 'Being called late after a family row to take sides. "Look at the bruise doctor".'

> 'A girl of 20 who wanted advice on how to change her career.'

Five per cent reported requests for prescriptions or medicines such as 'slimming tablets', 'a bottle of linctus for a head cold' for a 25-year-old man who said 'it's cheaper on the NHS'; and 'tranquillizers for mild anxiety.' Four per cent mentioned requests for unnecessary visits. Five per cent maintained: 'There is nothing trivial in any matter concerning the mental and physical welfare of the public.'

In the earlier study it was found that doctors who felt a high proportion of their consultations were trivial were less likely to have attended any courses in the last five years and were less likely to have direct access to hospital beds. They carried out relatively few procedures themselves and did not have access to many diagnostic facilities.

In the more recent study too, doctors with access to beds were comparatively unlikely to regard a high proportion of their consultations as trivial. So also were those who carried out several procedures themselves. But on the more recent study there was no clear association with the number of courses they had been on in the previous five years or with access to diagnostic facilities. Working in a partnership or health centre was not related to their estimates of the proportion of consultations they regarded as trivial but general practitioners who were trainers, those who were members of the Royal College of General Practitioners and those who did *not* use a deputizing service regarded relatively few of their consultations as trivial, inappropriate, or unnecessary. The figures are in *Table 31*.

One other characteristic of the doctors was clearly related to their estimates of the proportion of trivial consultations in 1977. The small number (24) of doctors who qualified in Asia thought on average that 53% of their consultations were for trivial, inappropriate, or unnecessary reasons. This compared with an average of 32% for doctors qualifying elsewhere. It is possible that doctors who have trained in countries where mortality and morbidity are much higher than in England and Wales may have a rather different threshold or definition for trivial complaints. But the implication is that in a sizeable proportion of consultations there is a wider disparity between them and their patients over their views of the general practitioner's role than for doctors who trained here or in Europe. There are more data about this in Chapter 7.

Doctors who enjoyed their work as a general practitioner very much tended to regard relatively few consultations as trivial: 58%

Table 31 'Trivial' consultations and some characteristics of the general practitioners and their work

	Proportion of doctors estimating that a quarter or more of their consultations were 'trivial'	*Estimated average proportion of 'trivial' consultations*	*No. of doctors (= 100%)*
Access to beds			
Yes	40%	29%	151
No	57%	36%	207
Score on procedures			
0–4	62%	38%	95
5 or more	46%	31%	262
Trainer			
Yes	32%	28%	31
No	52%	34%	323
Uses deputizing service			
Yes	60%	38%	158
No	42%	29%	199
Member of Royal College of General Practitioners			
Yes	24%	22%	68
No	57%	36%	291

thought a quarter or less fell into that category compared with 44% of those who said they enjoyed their work moderately and 17% of those who enjoyed it 'not very much' or 'not at all'. Feelings about the proportion of trivial consultations also related strongly to their views on conditions of work in the NHS, as can be seen from *Table 32*.

So for some general practitioners, feelings about trivial or inappropriate consultations inhibit their enjoyment of their work and colour their attitudes to the NHS – or vice versa. It may be that those doctors who are unsympathetic to the principle of free and open access to their services are more likely to perceive abuses. Does their attitude affect the way patients consult them and relate to them?

Table 32 Trivialities and views on conditions of work in the NHS

	Proportion of consultations felt to be 'trivial'					*All doctors*
	75% or more	*50% < 75%*	*25% < 50%*	*10% < 25%*	*Less than 10%*	
Views on conditions of work in NHS:	%	%	%	%	%	%
Very happy about them	—	—	1	5	12	4
Fairly happy about them	40	35	49	71	64	56
Rather unhappy	33	47	38	17	18	28
Very unhappy	27	18	12	5	6	11
Other comment	—	—	—	2	—	1
Number of general practitioners (= 100%)	30	57	93	110	67	363*

* Includes eight who did not answer the question about trivialities.

Table 33 Trivialities and patients' views and experiences

	Proportion of consultations felt to be 'trivial'				
	75% or more	*50% < 75%*	*25% < 50%*	*10% < 25%*	*Less than 10%*
Proportion of patients who regard their doctor as 'not so good' about taking time and not hurrying them	29%	25%	12%	13%	10%
Estimated annual consultation rate	2.9	3.9	4.1	3.3	3.7
Proportion of patients who had consulted their doctor in the last two weeks	5%	14%	10%	13%	19%
Number of patients (= 100%)	41	76	119	147	81

In 1977 there was a clear association between the proportion of patients who thought their doctor was 'not so good' about taking time and not hurrying them and the proportion of surgery consultations the doctor regarded as trivial, inappropriate, or unnecessary. This is shown in *Table 33*.

It is plausible that doctors who have a tendency to perceive consultations as trivial will seem impatient. And this could discourage patients from consulting them. In 1964 it appeared that patients of doctors who regarded a high proportion of their consultations as trivial had comparatively low consultation rates. In 1977 there was no association between doctors' views on the proportion of trivial, inappropriate, and unnecessary consultations and the number of consultations their patients reported in the previous twelve months (see *Table 32*). But there was a trend in the proportion reporting a consultation in the two weeks before interview, from 5% of those whose doctors thought at least three-quarters of their consultations were for trivial reasons to 19% of those whose doctors felt this about less than a tenth. So the evidence about this in the more recent study is equivocal, but there is certainly no evidence that high consultation rates among patients are associated with high proportions of 'trivial' consultations from the doctors' viewpoint. However, doctors who perceive themselves as being under pressure in that they described themselves as being more busy now than they had been ten years earlier reported a higher proportion of 'trivial' consultations, 36%, than those who thought they were less busy or there had been no change, 27%. Altogether two-thirds of the doctors said they felt 'more busy now.'

In general, the associations between patients' attitudes and behaviour and the views of their doctors about the proportion of trivial consultations are small. This is to be expected when we are not linking doctors' views on particular consultations with characteristics of patients.

The associations between doctors' characteristics or the circumstances of their practices and their estimates of 'trivial consultations' were more numerous and marked. It can be argued that trainers and members of the Royal College of General Practitioners are merely giving answers which they regard as more acceptable and that their responses do not necessarily reflect their 'real' views. Similarly doctors trained abroad could be *less* likely to be aware of the accepted response, while doctors with access to hospital beds might be *more* likely to know it. Even if a degree of sophistication contributes to this response it may extend to tolerance and labelling in the consultation. Doctors who feel it is inappropriate to record that they feel a high proportion of their consultations are 'trivial' may well become less likely to classify consultations in this way even to themselves.

In conclusion

It is clear from our data and from other studies that there has been no dramatic change in the rate at which patients consult their doctor, nor in the average list size, (see Ministry of Health 1965 and DHSS 1977b) while the amount of home visiting has declined. Yet many doctors said they felt more busy than they had been ten years before, and this feeling was associated with perceptions of a relatively high proportion of their consultations as being trivial, inappropriate, or unnecessary. At the same time doctors' estimates of the proportion of 'trivial' consultations had not changed between the two studies although most doctors thought that there was a growing tendency for people to seek help from doctors for problems in their family lives.

We feel that the main changes identified in this chapter are disappointing because there was no indication of a greater understanding between doctors and patients. Although most doctors felt that patients were generally more knowledgeable in 1977, this had not led to a reduction in the proportion of consultations that they regarded as trivial, inappropriate, or unnecessary. One source of this feeling about 'trivial' consultations seemed to be the seeking of advice about problems in peoples' family lives, since doctors who regarded this as inappropriate categorized a relatively high proportion of their consultations as 'trivial'. Over consultation about these family problems there was evidence of a possibly increasing area of conflict: fewer doctors in 1977 than in 1964 regarded it as appropriate although most of them in the later study felt that more patients were turning to them for this type of help.

From the patient's point of view there was evidence that the service had become more limited on two scores. More patients had come to feel that it was inappropriate to turn to their doctors for advice about problems such as children getting into trouble or difficulties between husband and wife, and doctors had become less willing to visit their homes.

One encouraging change for those who feel that too many medicines are prescribed was that patients had become less inclined to expect a prescription when they consulted their doctor and there was evidence that more patients felt their doctor was too inclined to prescribe.

4 Health centres

One of the most dramatic changes in general practice between 1964 and 1977 was the increase in health centres. Figures from the DHSS Annual Reports for 1976 and 1977 show that in 1965 there were 28 health centres and 215 general practitioners practising in them. By 1977 these figures had risen to 731 and 'about 3,800' respectively. So in the earlier study health centre practice was too insignificant to make separate analysis feasible or appropriate. By 1977 the position was quite different and it is possible to compare the experience and views of both doctors and patients in health centre practice with those in other types of practice. Sixteen per cent of the general practitioners who took part in our survey said they did all their general practitioner work in a health centre owned by an Area Health Authority. Another 6% said they did part of their work in one. Data from the DHSS about our sample of doctors give rather lower proportions, 13% having a main surgery in a health centre, 2% a branch surgery. The discrepancies, which were nearly all in the same direction, may be due, in part at any rate, to different dates to which the information refers. A third of the patients thought their doctor worked in a health centre, but it seems likely that many of them confused a privately owned or leased group practice with a health centre. However, if a doctor replied that he worked in a health centre no patient disagreed. The information from the doctors themselves has generally been used in the following analyses, and our comparisons are between those who work in a health centre at all and those who work entirely outside one. In looking at doctors' views of the advantages and disadvantages of health centres we have also considered the 15% of general practitioners who did not work in health centres at the time of the survey but said they would like to do so.

These comparisons give some clues about the extent to which some of the objectives of health centres have been achieved. So this chapter starts with a description of some of the aims of health centres that have been stated at various stages.

Some stated objectives of health centres

The Dawson Report on the Future Provision of Medical and Allied Services (1920) envisaged a primary health centre as 'an institution equipped for services of curative and preventive medicine to be conducted by the general practitioners of that district, in conjunction with an efficient nursing service and with the aid of visiting consultants and specialists.' It discussed the accommodation, equipment, and staffing of such centres and also maintained that:

> '.. it would be the home of . . . the intellectual life of the doctors of that unit. Those doctors, instead of being isolated as now from each other, would be brought together and in contact with consultants and specialists; there would develop an intellectual traffic and a camaraderie to the great advantage of the service.'

Although this report was 'quietly shelved within a few months of publication . . . in the long term it has been an immensely influential document' (Watkin 1975:111). Wofinden (1967) referred to the first trickle of health centres twenty years after the Dawson report which had become little more than a stream almost fifty years later: but he did feel there was 'a glimpse of the pent-up demand which, given the right encouragement from the Government, could develop into a broad, freely flowing river irrigating the desert of general medical practice and nourishing the growth of a co-ordinated medical service'! He held that: 'Social workers need to be based at health centres and work in the general practitioner team' and that 'the health visitor, home nurse and midwife should also be members of the team and be based at the centre.' He felt that: 'In the meantime, however, basing health visitors, midwives and home nurses at health centres does improve enormously their working relations with doctors, even though not wholly attached to the practice.' The

DHSS see another potential advantage of health centres – reducing demand on acute hospitals through the development of health care teams (DHSS 1976:17).

The Harvard Davis Report (1971) on the Organisation of Group Practice discussed the idea of holding consultative clinics in group practice centres and on balance concluded the advantages outweighed the disadvantages. They saw such sessions as being not only convenient but also reassuring for patients, promoting personal contact between hospital and community personnel with consequent opportunities for mutual education and professional improvement, fostering continuity and interdependence within the health service, and ensuring close collaboration between the consultant and the general practitioner. They quoted the experience of Wade and Elmes (1969) who demonstrated that out-patient sessions conducted in a health centre save the patient as much as two visits to the hospital.

So general practitioners working in health centres should have access to more appropriate equipment, they should have a closer and more satisfactory relationship with hospital doctors and with auxiliary staff, they should be more concerned with preventive medicine, and they should feel less isolated. In addition, health centres may reduce the demand on hospitals.

Before comparing the views and experiences of doctors and patients in and out of health centres it is relevant to ask whether health centres attract doctors with particular characteristics.

Which doctors?

Twenty-nine per cent of doctors under forty worked in a health centre compared with 20% of older doctors – but this difference might have arisen by chance and there was no general trend with the age of the doctor. However, doctors who worked in health centres were rather less likely to have been in general practice for twenty years or more, 38% of them compared with 52% of other doctors, and they were less likely to have been in the same practice that long, 23% against 37%.

Doctors who qualified in Great Britain were less likely to work in health centres than other doctors, 19% did so compared with 35% of doctors who qualified elsewhere. The country in which they qualified is shown for those working in health centres and for others in *Table 34*.

Table 34 Country of qualification and work in a health centre

	Doctors working in health centres		*All doctors*	*Proportion working in a health centre*
	Yes	*No*		
Country of qualification:	%	%	%	
Great Britain	72	85	83	19% (295)
N.Ireland	—	1	1 }	33% (27)
Eire	12	5	6 }	
Asia	10	6	7	33% (24)
Other	6	3	3	* (12)
Number of doctors (= 100%)	78	280	360	22% (362)

* Base number less than twenty.

The observation that a relatively high proportion of doctors who trained in Asia worked in a health centre is probably related to their short time in general practice. Only 9% of them had been in general practice for twenty or more years compared with 52% of doctors who qualified in other places.

The proportion of doctors working in health centres varied between our twenty study areas from none in Workington, Lambeth (Streatham), the City of Westminster, and Thanet to three-fifths in Shoreham and Burnley. It was not related in any systematic way to the density of an area nor did it vary significantly between constituencies with a Labour or a Conservative member of parliament.

There were relatively few, 6%, health centre practices among doctors working in restricted areas where further doctors are discouraged from practising. But the proportion among those working in designated areas, where Family Practitioner Committees are trying to encourage additional doctors was lower, 16%, than in 'open' areas where it was 33%.* These differences suggest that the policy of controls and incentives has been successful only in a negative way, keeping additional doctors out of the over-doctored areas but not in a positive way, by attracting them to the under-doctored areas (see Butler 1973).

* For a description of designated and restricted areas see Appendix I.

There were no significant differences between doctors working in health centres and others in their sex, qualifications, or membership of the Royal College of General Practitioners. There were however a number of differences in their type of practices and these are described next.

Type of practice

One difference associated with the relatively short time doctors who worked in health centres had been in the practice is that a comparatively small proportion of the patients on their list were aged 65 or more. (This is based on data from the DHSS about the doctors in our sample.) Twenty-eight per cent of doctors in health centres had less than 10% elderly patients compared with 14% of doctors working elsewhere. Health centres may be based on new estates or in new towns where there are few elderly people.

A number of other differences are summarized in *Table 35.* As expected, relatively few doctors working from a health centre, 4%,

Table 35 Health centres and type of practice

	Doctor works in health centre		*All doctors*
	Yes	*No*	
Average number of doctors in partnership*	3.2*	3.4*	3.4*
Single handed	4%	14%	12%
Has group practice allowance	83%	68%	71%
Doctor estimated that he/she was looking after 2,500 patients or more	77%	64%	67%
Average list size in practice 2,500 patients or more (DHSS data)	58%	45%	47%
Practice has:			
An ECG machine	53%	36%	40%
A refrigerator	97%	93%	94%
A microscope	37%	49%	46%
Treatment room	96%	71%	77%
Number of doctors (= 100%)	76	277	355

* Based only on doctors working in partnerships.

were single-handed. Among those working with others there was, however, no difference between health centre doctors and others in the number of doctors they worked with. Health centre doctors more often received a group practice allowance and they looked after rather more patients on average.

Doctors in health centres were more likely to have an ECG machine and a refrigerator in their practice but rather less likely to have a microscope. They were no more or less likely to have the other items of equipment we asked about – vaginal specula, haemoglobinometer, vision testing chart, peak flow meter, or vitallograph. And for doctors who did not have an ECG machine a desire for one was no greater or less among doctors working in a health centre than among other doctors.

There was no difference between health centre doctors and others in the proportions who said they had an appointment system for all their surgery consultations, 69%, for some, 20%, or for none, 11%.

Almost all doctors working from a health centre said there was a treatment room there compared with less than three-quarters of other doctors. And, as we will see next, they were more likely to work with a nurse.

Ancillary staff

As can be seen from *Table 36* doctors in health centres were more likely to have secretaries or receptionists who were employed by the Area Health Authority attached to the practice but they were rather less likely to employ secretaries or receptionists themselves. The average number of secretaries or receptionists working in the practice (that is, including both those who were attached and those who were employed) was similar, suggesting that attached secretaries or receptionists were an alternative to employed ones. The position in relation to nurses working in the surgery was rather different. Again doctors in health centre practices were more likely to have attached nurses and this meant that whereas almost all doctors in a health centre worked with a nurse of some kind, one in five of those working elsewhere did not.

The type of work undertaken by nurses working in a health centre was rather different from that of nurses in other types of practice. In general the scope of the nurses' work seemed greater in health centres where patients were more likely to have direct access to the

Table 36 Health centres and ancillary staff

	Doctor works in health centre		All doctors
	Yes	No	
Practice has:			
Attached secretaries/receptionists	33%	12%	17%
Employed secretaries/receptionists	78%	94%	90%
Average number of secretaries/ receptionists attached or employed	4.2	4.1	4.1
Attached nurses*	90%	61%	67%
Employed nurses*	30%	37%	35%
Either employed or attached nurses*	99%	80%	84%
Other attached staff:			
Health visitors	97%	85%	88%
Midwives	92%	78%	80%
Social workers	38%	18%	23%
Nurse seeing patient entirely outside surgery	64%	47%	51%
Number of doctors (=100%)	75	275	351

* Nurses working at least part of their time in the surgery.

Table 37 Health centres and the work of nurses

	Doctor works in health centre		All doctors with a nurse at surgery
	Yes	No	
Nurse at surgery sometimes:			
Stitches cuts	28%	14%	18%
Syringes ears	92%	77%	81%
Patient has direct access to nurses	79%	65%	70%
Nurse frequently does things that patients would otherwise have to go to hospital for	47%	34%	38%
Number of doctors working in practice with an attached or employed nurse at surgery (=100%)	78	224	304

nurse and where the nurses more often stitched cuts and syringed ears themselves. The comparisons, based only on practices with a nurse, are in *Table 37*. Possibly related to this the doctors in health centres more often reckoned that the nurses frequently did things that the patient would otherwise have to go to hospital for, but they did not think nurses were any more likely to do things that the doctors would otherwise have to do. (Fifty-eight per cent of doctors in practices with a nurse thought the nurse did this frequently, 36% occasionally, 6% never.) The more frequent existence of a treatment room at health centres probably contributed to these differences. But when only practices with a treatment room are considered nurses were still more likely to stitch cuts and syringe ears when they worked at health centres. The other differences were also in the same direction but no longer reached a level of statistical significance.

Other types of attached staff were also more common at health centres than at other types of practice. If doctors worked in a practice without attached home nurses those in health centres were no more or less likely to want such a nurse – one in six of them wanted this, but doctors in health centres were more likely to want a social worker: 65% of doctors at a health centre where there was no attached social worker wanted one, compared with 47% of doctors working elsewhere. This may be related to differences in their views on the appropriate role of the general practitioner, discussed later in this chapter.

Up to now we have concentrated on the differences between the staffing and organization of doctors working in health centres and those of other doctors. But the lack of differences between the two groups is also illuminating. They did not differ in the extent to which they used a deputizing service nor in the average number of nights a week they were on call. So the organization in a health centre did not give doctors more free nights, neither did it mean that patients less often had a completely strange doctor in an emergency. Their practices were no more or less likely to have trainees or to take medical students on a regular basis. The greater number of attached staff in health centres did not appear to have improved their communications with the social services. A quarter of general practitioners described these as 'good', just over two-fifths as 'fair', and a third as 'poor'. What of relationships with the hospital?

Hospital and other professional relationships

Doctors who worked in a health centre were relatively *un*likely to have a hospital appointment, 30% of them had one against 43% of other doctors. Was this because those in health centres obtained their professional contacts with their colleagues there and were therefore less likely to seek a hospital appointment? Apparently not. More of those in health centres said they would like to have a hospital appointment, 33% compared with 21% of other doctors. Similar proportions of both groups, just over a third, did not have one and did not want one. They did not differ in their access to hospital beds, nor in their desire for these.

Criticisms about inadequate consultation with general practitioners over the admission and discharge of patients to and from hospital were made with equal frequency by doctors working in health centres and others. Only a minority of general practitioners, a fifth, felt that consultation over admission was inadequate, but two-thirds regarded consultation about discharge as unsatisfactory. So there is no evidence here of a closer or more satisfactory link with hospital colleagues for doctors working in health centres.

When doctors were asked to rate the relative importance to them in keeping up-to-date of the various sources listed in *Table 38* doctors

Table 38 Relative importance of different ways of keeping up-to-date for health centre doctors and others

	Average rank*		
	Doctor works in health centre		*All doctors*
	Yes	*No*	
Professional meetings	2.3	2.3	2.3
Informal discussion with other doctors	3.4	3.0	3.0
Drughouse literature or representatives	4.6	4.4	4.5
Journals, books, and other publications	2.4	2.7	2.6
Courses	2.3	2.6	2.6
Number of doctors	70	242	313

*1 = high, 5 = low.

who worked in health centres rated informal discussion with other doctors as being of rather less importance. This is a rather surprising finding. If doctors in health centres have more frequent contact with professional colleagues does this lead to a disregarding or an underestimation of the value of such contacts?

Doctors working in health centres ranked courses more highly than doctors who did not work in a health centre but if anything they had been on fewer courses in the last five years than had other doctors: 17% of them said they had been on less than five compared with 8% of other doctors.

Attendance at courses or professional meetings and informal discussions with other doctors may be useful ways of keeping up-to-date but we have no measure of the extent to which they achieved this. We do however know something about their attitudes, which may be related to their professional contacts.

Doctors' attitudes

When asked whether they thought partnerships, trainees, appointment systems, and deputizing services an advantage or disadvantage to doctors and to patients, doctors working in health centres did not differ from others in their replies. Doctors working in health centres were rather less likely to see medical students as an advantage to doctors: 37% thought this compared with 53% of other doctors. (On balance partnerships and appointment systems were seen as an advantage both to patients and doctors; trainees, medical students, and deputizing services were seen as more of an advantage to doctors than to patients. The figures are given elsewhere.)

The similarity of the opinions of health centre doctors and others on these topics is not surprising in view of the similarity of their practices in these respects. Rather more surprisingly, since more doctors in health centres had changed their practice in the last ten years, they made similar estimates as other doctors about changes over the last ten years in consultation rates, home visiting, patients' knowledge of disease, and the relative prestige of general practitioners in the community and in the profession. But as can be seen from *Table 39* a higher proportion of doctors in health centres thought that patients were now more likely to question whether the doctor was right than they were ten years ago. Later in this chapter

Table 39 Health centres and doctors' views

	Doctor works in health centre		*All doctors*
	Yes	*No*	
General practitioner:			
Thinks patients now more likely to question whether doctor is right than they were ten years ago	71%	53%	57%
In future would like to see more emphasis on:			
Team approach	65%	44%	49%
Health education	86%	76%	78%
Thinks it is appropriate for people to seek help from their general practitioner with problems in their family lives	57%	70%	67%
Would like an attached social worker	65%*	47%*	49%*
Number of doctors (=100%)	79	283	365

* Based only on doctors without an attached social worker.

it will be shown that age, sex, and social class variations between patients in the two groups cannot account for this difference.

The doctors did not differ in their estimates of the proportion of their surgery consultations which they felt to be trivial, inappropriate, or unnecessary. Neither did doctors in health centres and others differ in their views about the emphasis they would like to see in the future on home visiting in general practice or on community rather than hospital care. But the doctors in health centres wanted to see more emphasis than other doctors on a team approach and on health education.

Another difference was that doctors in health centres were less likely than other doctors to think that it was appropriate for people to seek help from their general practitioner for problems in their family lives. Initially it was thought that it might link up with their views on team care and on the role of the social worker in general practice, as doctors in health centres were both more likely to have a social worker attached to their practice and to want one if they did not have one. But when the comparison between health centre doctors and others was confined to doctors who qualified in Great Britain the difference in their views about consultation for family problems disappeared.

A disappointing finding was that the investment in health centres did not seem to have led to more satisfied doctors. There was no difference between doctors working in health centres and others in the extent to which they said they enjoyed their work as a general practitioner, nor in their satisfaction with their conditions of work in the National Health Service. What of their perceptions of the advantages and disadvantages of working in a health centre?

Doctors' perceptions of the advantages and disadvantages of health centres

The most frequently perceived advantages of working in a health centre were the facilities available and the contact with other health workers.* These were seen with equal frequency by those who already worked in a health centre and by those who wanted to do so, less often by those who did not want to work in one (see *Table 40*). Over a third of those who wanted to work in one saw reduced responsibility for administration as an advantage, but only 4% of those already working in one felt this, so this may be an illusory attraction. One in seven of all general practitioners mentioned contact or increased contact with general practice colleagues or hospital staff and the possibilities of a second opinion as an advantage of working in a health centre.

In terms of the disadvantages, shown in *Table 41,* the possible political constraints may be the main deterrent for those who do not want to go into one. High costs were more often seen as a disadvantage by those who worked in one or wanted to do so than by others. Fears of a deteriorating doctor-patient relationship were not borne out by those with experience of the situation.

* 'What, if any, do you see as the main advantages of working in a health centre?'

Table 40 Perceived advantages of working in a health centre

	General practitioners who:			*All general practi-tioners*
	Work in a health centre	*Would like to work in one*	***Would not** like to work in one*	
	%	%	%	%
Facilities: better equipment; economies of scale; available under one roof; space; modern; purpose-built building; more comfortable for patients	56	53	19	32
Contact with other health workers; availability of ancillary staff	55	53	21	32
Contact or increased contact with GP colleagues or hospital staff; possibilities of second opinion	17	21	11	14
Professional contact (unspecified who with); reduction in GP isolation (unspecified why)	7	3	6	6
Reduced responsibility for administration; freedom from organizing maintenance, staffing, servicing, etc. of building	4	37	12	13
Financial: reduced cost; no initial capital expenditure on furniture, fittings; shared costs for new equipment	17	11	12	13
Distribution of work load: arranging off-duty, holiday rotas	1	11	7	6
Better accommodation —unspecified	1	3	1	1
Efficiency	3	11	2	3
Other	12	5	3	6
None	4	—	43	28
Number of general practitioners (= 100%)	75	38	207	336

Table 41 Perceived disadvantages of working in a health centre

	General practitioners who:			*All general practitioners*
	Work in a health centre	*Would like to work in one*	*Would not like to work in one*	
Possible political constraints:	%	%	%	%
loss of professional independence; no security of tenure; problems of not owning building; possible eviction	23	34	41	36
Lack of personal control over working conditions:				
administrative interference in day-to-day running; bureaucracy, inflexibility regimentation of organization; no control over staffing	36	21	36	34
Impersonal atmosphere:				
loss of homely atmosphere, noise, size, and complexity for patients	18	24	27	24
Costs:				
high/increased running costs; difficulty in regulating/controlling costs	26	26	14	19
Doctor-patient relationship:				
deterioration of individual relationship, loss of continuity of contact with individual patient	3	5	19	14
Distance:				
Problems for patients travelling to centralized surgeries	4	11	5	5
Problems of cooperation/compatibility:				
with other general practitioners	4	3	3	3
with other staff in health centre	4	—	2	3
with colleagues unspecified	3	—	2	2
Other	29	—	14	16
None	14	11	1	5
Number of general practitioners (=100%)	73	38	207	334

When it comes to making a general assessment, those who worked in health centres and those who wanted to do so were much more likely than the others to see health centres as an advantage for both patients and doctors. And those who wanted to go into one were, if anything, rather more optimistic about the advantages of a health centre for both patients and doctors than those already working in one – but the differences between those two groups, shown in *Table 42,* might have occurred by chance, except that significantly more of those working in one saw it as a disadvantage from the point of view of the doctor.

Table 42 Health centres seen as an advantage or disadvantage for patients and doctors?

	General practitioners who:			*All general practitioners*
	Work in a health centre	*Would like to work in one*	*Would not like to work in one*	
For patients	%	%	%	%
An advantage	64	70	10	30
A disadvantage	9	8	54	37
Equally balanced	26	20	35	32
Other comment	1	2	1	1
For doctors	%	%	%	%
An advantage	59	75	12	31
A disadvantage	15	3	64	44
Equally balanced	25	20	23	24
Other comment	1	2	1	1
Number of general practitioners (= 100%)	78	40	218	354

Patients and their views

Among the patients in our sample there was no clear trend with age in the proportion whose doctor worked in a health centre and similar proportions of patients under and over the age of 65 had such a doctor. Neither were there any differences over this between men and women, nor between patients of different social classes. So, basic demographic differences of patients cannot account for any variations in patients' views or in the doctor-patient relationship although, as noted earlier, the doctors in health centres had a relatively low proportion of elderly patients according to DHSS records.

In addition, and perhaps more surprisingly, there were no significant differences between health centre patients and others in the length of time they said they had had their doctor. But a higher proportion of health centre patients said their doctor had moved since they started going to him, 32% compared with 14%.* And rather fewer patients in health centres said they had 'inherited' their doctor when he took over from another one, 33% against 41%.*

While patients at health centres had been with their present doctor for as long as other patients they were less likely to feel that they knew their doctor very well. Twenty-eight per cent of them said they did not know their doctor well, compared with 19% of patients whose doctor did not work in a health centre. This difference did not arise because they consulted their general practitioner less frequently or because they less often had a home visit. However, patients at health centres were more likely than others to see their doctor's partners or colleagues as much or more than their own doctor: 33% against 20% had done this within the last twelve months.

In spite of not knowing their doctor so well patients at health centres were no less likely than others to regard their doctor as something of a personal friend, or to say they would consult him or her about a personal problem. They were also as likely to regard a general practitioner as an appropriate person to talk to about problems such as children getting into trouble or difficulties between husband and wife although, as we showed earlier, doctors in health centres themselves were less likely to feel it appropriate for people to

* These proportions are based on patients' statements about whether or not their doctor worked in a health centre.

seek help from their general practitioners for problems in their family lives.

It might have been expected that patients going to health centres would regard their doctor's surgery as well equipped and up-to-date and the waiting room as pleasant and comfortable. In practice there was no difference in patients' assessments of these facilities but of course patients may have higher expectations when they go to a health centre. A higher proportion of patients attending health centres said they had waited for an hour or more at their last consultation: 16% against 5%. (It will be recalled that similar proportions of health centre doctors and others had an appointment system.) And patients attending health centres were more critical of their doctor about the times they were kept waiting: 30% compared with 17% said their doctor was 'not so good' about this. Fewer health centre patients also felt their doctor was 'good' about visiting when asked: 61% against 71%, but there was no difference between the two groups in their views about receptionists being helpful or unhelpful.

There were also one or two ways in which direct doctor-patient relationships seemed rather less good in health centres. Patients in health centres were less likely to regard their doctor as easy to talk to* (69% compared with 83%) and more of them were critical of him or her about explaining things (30% against 19%). They were no more – or less – critical of their doctor about examining people carefully and thoroughly, taking time and not hurrying them and listening to what they said.

Patients whose doctors worked in a health centre were no more or less likely to say they would go to a general practitioner rather than the hospital if they cut their leg at home so that it needed stitching. A fifth of both groups said they would go to their general practitioner. (The time patients estimated that it took them to get to their doctor's surgery was also similar for the two groups.) When asked if they would expect their doctor (or the nurse) to cope with a small cyst that needed cutting out, or to send them to hospital, there was no difference in the expectations of health centre patients and others over this, nor in the women patients' expectations about referral for a vaginal examination. But fewer patients at health

* 'And would you say it is easy to talk to your doctor and ask him questions or do you feel it is not possible to talk to him as much as you'd like?'

centres expected their doctor to refer them to hospital for a blood test rather than to have it done at the surgery: 24% compared with 34% for non-health centre patients, and more health centre patients reported that a general practitioner or practice nurse had taken a specimen of blood or urine from them during the last twelve months: 35% against 18%. However, patients attending health centres were no less likely than patients from other types of practice to have been to hospital as an out-patient in the previous twelve months, and if anything a rather *higher* proportion of them said they had been admitted to hospital as an in-patient, 15% compared with 8% of other patients.

How far can some of the differences in patients' attitudes and experiences be accounted for by differences in the doctors rather than in whether or not they work at a health centre?

In a later chapter we will see that patients tended to be more critical of doctors who did not qualify in Great Britain over a number of issues. And this seems to contribute to the higher level of criticism of doctors in health centres about explaining things or being easy to talk to. If the comparisons are confined to doctors who qualified in Great Britain the proportion who said their doctor was not easy to talk to was 25% of health centre patients, 15% of others, and the proportions who felt the doctor was not so good about explaining things were 26% and 18% respectively. In both cases the differences were still in the same direction but had dropped below the level of statistical significance. This suggests that it is not the inherent nature of health centre practice which leads to more criticism among patients.

In conclusion

Other studies have concluded that the great majority of health centres fail to realize their potential in terms of promoting the primary health care team and encouraging better working relationships between the various workers (Beales 1978). And the most striking finding from this study is the relative lack of difference between doctors working in health centres and elsewhere.

Doctors in health centres were rather more likely to work in a health care team with other types of professionals, and nurses in health centres had a somewhat wider scope of work and worked more independently than nurses in other practices, but the differences were not large and in many aspects of their work there was little or no difference between the two groups.

Although a majority of doctors working in them saw health centres as an advantage for both patients and doctors, the doctors themselves did not report enjoying their work any more if they were based in a health centre. And even more disappointingly for the advocates of health centres, there is little or no evidence that patients have benefitted from them, and some indication that, if anything, doctor-patient relationships are rather less good in health centres than elsewhere.

5 Working together

The increase in partnerships and health centres is associated with a greater emphasis on team care. But the impetus towards team care comes from other sources too. Reedy (1977) sees the concept of primary care delivered by a team of health workers as having developed in this way:

> 'As more specialised knowledge and increasing access to the technology of medical investigation became available to general practitioners, it was inevitable that they would seek to shed lower status activities and widen their spheres of competence and influence.'

This chapter is concerned not with the dynamics of team care (that would need a different sort of study) but with the main sorts of people patients may encounter when they go to see their doctor at the surgery. So it is the roles of the secretaries or receptionists, nurses, social workers, medical students, and trainees which are examined in this chapter. The work of health visitors and midwives, who may be important members of a team, are not considered in any detail because they tend to be concerned with particular groups of patients and much of their work is in patients' homes and specialized clinics.

Secretaries and receptionists

All but four doctors, 1%, said they had a secretary or receptionist in 1977 compared with a quarter who did not have one in 1964. (Three of the four without one in 1977 were single-handed; none of them employed a nurse either but two had attached nurses who did some work at the surgery.) In a previous chapter we saw that the average number of secretaries attached to or employed by a practice was four, and this number rose from two for single-handed doctors to over six for those in practices with five or more doctors. Most practices, nine out of ten, employed secretaries or receptionists directly but roughly one in five had attached secretaries employed by the AHA. With the increase in the number of secretaries and receptionists there has developed a picture of them as seeing their main role as being to protect the doctor from importunate patients (see Stimson and Webb 1975: 114–18).

One way in which they might perform a gate-keeping function is by asking patients why they want to see the doctor. Doctors with secretaries or receptionists were asked if they liked the receptionists to ask patients who came to see the doctor at the surgery why they wanted to do so. Fifteen per cent said they liked them to do this routinely, another 23% said they liked them to do this occasionally, 40% said for emergencies only, and 22% said they did not like them to do this ever. Information from patients gives a similar picture: 19% of those who had had any contact with a secretary or receptionist said she always asked them why they wanted to see the doctor, 18% that she sometimes did so, and 57% that she had never done so. (Three per cent did not know and 3% said they always told her anyway.)

Rather more general practitioners who worked in small practices with one or two doctors said they liked the receptionists to ask patients routinely why they wanted to see the doctor at the surgery, 21% of them did so compared with 11% of doctors in larger partnerships. Possibly the doctors in the smaller groups have a closer relationship with their receptionists and feel they can supervise them better or trust their judgement more.

Patients were less likely to regard receptionists as helpful if they asked them why they wanted to see the doctor. Altogether 49% of patients described receptionists as 'very helpful' and this proportion was 53% if they never asked, 45% if they did so sometimes, and 36% if they always did so. This was in spite of the fact that most of the patients who were ever asked, three-quarters, felt the receptionist asked 'the right amount.' But one in five thought she asked too much. Some comments were:

'It's between your doctor and yourself. Someone asking you why you want to see the doctor leads you at times not to make an appointment, not to go. It's intimidating and shouldn't happen.'

'I tell them quite politely "Are you qualified? Are you the doctor?" She's only there to push a pen and file the cards.'

The majority, 70%, of those who said the receptionist always asked why they wanted to see the doctor said they did not mind, one in ten said it depended, one in five disliked it.

A higher proportion of those who were not asked why they wanted to see the doctor were opposed to the idea, 30%.

'It's embarrassing enough having to go to the doctor without having to tell someone else about it – It is for me because I have to pluck up courage to go to the doctor – and to have to relate it twice!'

'Because she's not the doctor. She thinks she is at times. She seems to think she can run it on her own. She's very disliked, but very efficient.'

A fifth of those who were ever asked why they wanted to see the doctor said they felt receptionists were making it difficult for them to see the doctor. Only 3% of other patients and 6% of all patients felt this.

The doctors who liked receptionists to ask routinely why patients want to see them regarded a relatively high proportion of their consultations as trivial, inappropriate, or unnecessary: they estimated that an average of 48% fell into those categories compared with with an average of 30% among other doctors.

The evidence from this study suggests that when receptionists asked patients why they wanted to see the doctor, this created a barrier between patients and doctors and discouraged some people from consulting the doctor. The proportion who had not consulted at all in the last twelve months was 27% among those who said the receptionists always asked about this, 18% among those who said the receptionists never or only sometimes did so, while the proportions who had consulted five or more times were 18% and 32% in the two groups.*

* There was no difference between those who said the receptionist sometimes asked and those who said she never did. If the difference

However 72% of all patients felt that receptionists were helping them to get to the doctor and this proportion was still 64% among those who said the receptionists always asked why they wanted to see the doctor. But if patients usually had to wait three days or more to get an appointment when they wanted one as soon as possible only 42% thought the receptionists were helping them to see the doctor compared with 80% if they could get an appointment within 24 hours.

Nurses in the surgery

The proportion of doctors who had a nurse working in the practice increased from 12% in 1964 to 84% in 1977. In the recent study two-thirds had an attached nurse employed by the Area Health Authority who worked at least part of her time at the surgery, a third of the doctors employed a nurse directly, a fifth had both an employed and an attached nurse. In addition, half the doctors said they had a nurse attached to their practice who worked entirely outside their surgery.* Taking all these different working arrangements into account only 7% of doctors did not have either sort of nurse attached to or employed by their practices.

In their national study in 1974 Reedy, Philips, and Newell (1976) found that practices with an attached nurse were *more* likely to employ one; 26.4% did so compared with 20.0% of those without an attached nurse. They did not distinguish between attached nurses working in the surgery and those working entirely outside. A comparable analysis on our data, but based on doctors rather than practices, showed an insignificant difference in the opposite direction (the proportions were 34% and 43%). But if we consider only attached nurses doing some or all of their work at the surgery we find that doctors in practices with attached nurses were *less* likely to employ nurses: 27% of them did so against 52% of those without

---

between the 'always' and 'sometimes' had arisen because those who consulted frequently had more experience and therefore were aware that receptionists did not always do the same thing, then we would also have expected a higher rate of consultation among the 'sometimes' than among those who said the receptionists never asked.

* 'Are any of these *attached* to your practice but not employed by you: health visitors, midwives, social workers, nurses seeing patients entirely outside your surgery?'

an attached nurse. This suggests that attached nurses working in the surgery are sometimes used as a substitute for employed nurses, although later on we will show that the work they do differs in a number of ways.

The rest of this section is about nurses working at the surgery.

Half the general practitioners who worked on their own had neither an attached nurse nor an employed nurse at the surgery and this proportion dropped to 19% of those in partnerships of two, and 4% in partnerships of five or more. (The proportions with attached nurses and with employed nurses by size of partnership were shown in Chapter 2.)

Associated with this trend, older doctors were less likely to have a nurse working in their practice surgery; 76% of those aged 60 or more were in practices with a surgery nurse, compared with 96% of those under 40.

Table 43 Variations in doctors' equipment with the presence of a nurse at the surgery

	Doctor in practice with:				
	Attached nurse only at surgery	*Employed nurse only*	*Both attached and employed nurse*	*Either sort of nurse*	*No nurse*
Doctor in practice that has:					
Refrigerator	94%	94%	99%	95%	86%
Vaginal speculum	98%	100%	100%	99%	98%
ECG machine	37%	60%	49%	44%	17%
Haemoglobinometer	32%	47%	42%	37%	28%
Vision testing chart	99%	98%	97%	98%	93%
Peak flow meter or vitallograph	80%	73%	82%	79%	67%
A microscope	40%	52%	63%	47%	41%
Number of doctors (= 100%)	176	62	67	305	58

Another clear difference between practices with a surgery nurse and those without one was in the existence of a treatment room. Less than a third of the doctors, 29%, without a surgery nurse had one, whereas 86% of those who had such a nurse also had a treatment room. In addition those with a nurse had rather more equipment. This can be seen from *Table 43*.

Doctors who estimated that they looked after a relatively small number of NHS patients were no more or less likely to work in practices with an employed or an attached nurse. Nine-tenths of the doctors in practices that employed a nurse said the patients had direct access to the nurse, but only about half of them said that as a matter of policy the nurse sometimes made the first contact for an

Table 44 Direct access to and first contacts with the nurse

	Doctor in practice with:			
	Attached nurse only at surgery	*Employed nurse only*	*Both attached and employed nurse*	*Either sort of nurse*
At surgery patients have direct access to a nurse:	%	%	%	%
Yes	54	90	93	70
No	45	10	7	29
Other comment	1	—	—	1
Doctor said that as a matter of policy the nurse sometimes makes first contact for an episode of illness:				
In surgery	%	%	%	%
Yes	19	56	49	33
No	81	44	51	67
In patient's home	%	%	%	%
Yes	13	7	12	12
No	87	93	88	88
Number of doctors (= 100%)	173	60	67	301

episode of illness. The apparent discrepancy may arise because patients tend to go directly to a nurse for various services such as dressings and for follow-up consultations, but as a matter of policy about half the doctors always preferred to be the first contact for an episode of illness. Patients were less likely to have direct access to an attached nurse and a smaller proportion of doctors thought it was appropriate for such a nurse to make the first contact for an episode of illness at the surgery. On the question of first contacts by nurses in patients' homes, relatively few doctors, one in eight of those with a nurse, thought this was appropriate but the difference between those with attached and those with employed nurses was, if anything, in the opposite direction. The figures are in *Table 44*.

Doctors were asked whether their attached or employed nurses ever did any of the things listed in *Table 45* at the surgery.

Table 45 Nurses' activities at the surgery

	Doctor in practice with:			
	Attached nurse only at surgery	*Employed nurse only*	*Both attached and employed nurse*	*Either sort of nurse*
	%	%	%	%
Syringe ears	73	93	90	81
Assist at vaginal exams	53	80	93	67
Take blood	45	57	69	53
Stitch cuts	14	28	21	18
Open abscesses	6	26	18	13
Excise cysts	1	3	3	2
Fit IUDs	—	2	3	1
None of these	16	2	1	10
Number of doctors (=100%)	176	61	67	304

Employed nurses carried out more procedures than attached ones, but attached nurses were more likely to carry out procedures when there was a treatment room. The proportions are shown in *Table 46*.

Table 46 Activities of attached nurses by whether there was a treatment room at the surgery

	Treatment room	
	Yes	*No*
	%	%
Syringe ears	80	41
Assist at vaginal exams	56	34
Take blood	51	22
Stitch cuts	15	6
Open abscesses	8	—
Excise cysts	1	—
Fit IUDs	—	—
None of these	11	41
Number of doctors with attached nurses only (= 100%)	142	32

So few doctors with an employed nurse did not have a treatment room, 9%, that it is not possible to do a comparable analysis for them.

How did the presence of a nurse affect the doctors' own activities? The general practitioners were asked whether they personally undertook a number of procedures in their practice 'more often than not', 'occasionally', or 'never' when they arose. Replies are shown in *Table 47*.

Two consistent differences with the various procedures were that doctors undertook the procedures themselves more often if there was either sort of nurse than if there was no nurse at all and they were also more likely to do them if there was an employed nurse than if there was an attached nurse. If the doctors have answered our questions correctly nurses are more likely to undertake a procedure if the doctor does it himself or herself, and vice versa. This is demonstrated directly for stitching cuts and taking blood in *Table 48*. At first this might seem a surprising finding – why keep a dog and bark yourself? But reflection suggests it is a reasonable one. In practices where patients have their cuts stitched and blood taken on the spot, without referral to hospital, both doctors and nurses are likely to be involved in the procedure. The nurse presumably does more because she copies the doctor and is supported and feels safer because it is a 'usual' activity in the practice.

Table 47 Variations in doctors' activities with the presence of a nurse at the surgery

Doctor personally undertakes these procedures when they arise:	*Doctor in practice with:*				*All doctors*
	Attached nurse only at surgery	*Employed nurse only*	*Both attached and employed nurse*	*No nurse*	
Fits IUDs	%	%	%	%	%
More often than not	27	46	43	7	30
Occasionally	6	10	12	17	9
Never	67	44	45	76	61
Excises simple cysts	%	%	%	%	%
More often than not	26	40	45	9	29
Occasionally	39	39	32	36	37
Never	35	21	23	55	34
Takes blood	%	%	%	%	%
More often than not	55	74	52	38	55
Occasionally	43	23	46	53	42
Never	2	3	2	9	3
Stitches cuts	%	%	%	%	%
More often than not	39	71	48	22	43
Occasionally	47	18	43	57	43
Never	14	11	9	21	14
Examines vagina with speculum	%	%	%	%	%
More often than not	84	87	94	66	83
Occasionally	14	11	6	31	15
Never	2	2	—	3	2
Average procedure score	5.5	6.4	6.1	4.5	5.6
Number of doctors (=100%)	175	61	66	58	362

Table 48 The relationship between the doctors and nurses stitching cuts and taking blood

	Doctor in practice with:		
	A nurse who stitches cuts	*A nurse who does not stitch cuts*	*No nurse*
Doctor personally stitches cuts:	%	%	%
More often than not	74	42	22
Occasionally	20	45	58
Never	6	13	20
Number of doctors (=100%)	54	249	59
	A nurse who takes blood	*A nurse who does not take blood*	*No nurse*
Doctor personally takes blood:	%	%	%
More often than not	65	52	37
Occasionally	33	45	54
Never	2	3	9
Number of doctors (=100%)	159	144	59

Reverting to the difference between employed and attached nurses we found that more of the doctors with employed nurses than of those with attached nurses felt that the nurse(s) in their practice frequently did things that they or their partner would otherwise do if there was not a nurse: 75% of those with an employed nurse felt this compared with 45% of those with only an attached nurse. They were also more likely to think that the nurse often did things that patients would otherwise have to go to hospital for if there was not a nurse. The figures are in *Table 49*. Our data from patients show that 35% of those whose doctor worked with a nurse had attended an out-patient's department in the previous year, compared with 41% of other patients – an insignificant difference.

To what extent were doctors' views related to the presence or absence of a nurse at the surgery? Nearly all the doctors working in a practice with some type of nurse thought that having a nurse at the

Table 49 The nurse as an alternative to the doctor or the hospital

	Doctor in practice with:			
	Attached nurse only at surgery	*Employed nurse only*	*Both attached and employed nurse*	*Either sort of nurse*
Doctor estimated that the nurse did things at the surgery:				
that the doctor or his partners would otherwise do if there was not a nurse	%	%	%	%
Frequently	45	77	73	57
Occasionally	45	18	27	36
Never	10	5	—	7
that patients would otherwise have to go to hospital for if there was not a nurse	%	%	%	%
Frequently	29	49	49	38
Occasionally	42	33	37	39
Never	29	18	14	23
Number of doctors (=100%)	176	61	67	304

surgery was an advantage to patients (95% thought that) and to doctors (94%). Rather fewer of those without a nurse held those views but even among them the majority thought a nurse was an advantage to patients (80%) and to doctors (82%). Having a nurse was not related to their estimates of the proportion of surgery consultations which they regarded as trivial, inappropriate, or unnecessary. And those without a nurse did not enjoy their work as a general practitioner any less – or more – than those with one. Perhaps surprisingly having a nurse did not appear to affect the emphasis they would like to see on a team approach in general practice in the future. Possibly those who already had a nurse did not see a need for a greater emphasis on a team approach.* Nor did they differ in the emphasis they would like to see on community care, on health education, or on home visiting nor on the importance they attached to continuity of care. But doctors *without* a nurse attached more importance to family care, 41% of them regarding it as 'very important' compared with 24% of doctors working in a practice with a nurse at the surgery. Part of this difference arose because older doctors were more likely to believe in family care and less likely to have a nurse but among younger doctors, under 40, the difference remained. Finally, having a nurse at the surgery did not seem to affect doctors' views on communications with social services – 24% described them as 'good', 44% as 'fair', and 32% as 'poor'.

Turning now to patients' views and experiences. Patients were more aware of employed than of attached nurses possibly because of differences in the amount of time they spend at the surgery. If the doctor had an employed nurse 61% of the patients realized this, 18% did not know, and 21% thought there was no nurse. Corresponding proportions when the doctor had an attached nurse only were 29% reporting that there was a nurse at the surgery, 22% saying they did not know, and 49% saying there was not one. Only 4% of patients with doctors who said they did not have a surgery nurse thought there was one. And of course changes over time would lead to some discrepancies.

Patients who thought there was a nurse working at the surgery were asked what sort of things she did or advised about. Dressings were mentioned by 49%, injections by 44%, ear syringing by 19%, blood tests by 12%, weighing by 8%, and other things including vaccinations and immunizations by 35%. Sixteen per cent said they did not know. Just under a third, 31%, of patients who said there was a nurse at the surgery said she had done something for them in the last twelve months. This meant that 14% of patients who had consulted a doctor in the last twelve months had received some help or care from the nurse. Of those who had been helped by the nurse, 19% had had their ears syringed, 17% dressings or stitchings, 14% blood tests, another 14% immunizations or vaccinations for

* The question asked: 'Thinking about the future development of health care, would you like to see more or less emphasis on the team approach in general practice?'

flu, tetanus, etc., and a similar proportion had been chaperoned or helped with an internal examination, smear test, or fitting an IUD. Eight per cent had been given injections, 7% antenatal care, 5% had received front-line care before they saw the doctor, 3% had been visited at home, and 13% had other types of care. Some descriptions of what the nurse did and how the patient felt about it were:

> 'My finger nail – she pierced a hole in it to release the pressure. I felt better with her doing it, being a nurse. A doctor's for finding out what's wrong with you (doctors in hospital are for operating) and it seems natural for a nurse to do that sort of thing.'
>
> 'She took a blood test. I felt more confident than going to the hospital.'
>
> 'A cancer smear. I was a bit nervous and embarrassed because I knew her. She was a neighbour.'
>
> 'She syringed my ears out. Alright – they get experience. I took it in my stride. They're there to help you and if you get grumpy about it that's your look out.'

Nurses seemed to be seeing a broad spectrum of patients. Expressing the number who said they had had some treatment from the nurse in the last twelve months as a proportion of all patients who had consulted the doctor during that time, there were no significant variations with age or sex.

There was some indication that patients in practices with a nurse (as reported by the doctor) may have consulted their doctor slightly more often than those in practices without one. The estimated annual consultation rates in the two groups were 3.8 and 3.0 respectively – a difference which might have occurred by chance. And the proportions who had consulted their doctor ten or more times were 14% of those in practices with a nurse, 7% in those without one. So a nurse may lead to more frequent attendance. This conclusion is supported by data about consultations in the two weeks before the interview. From these data the estimated annual consultation rate was 4.6 for those in practices with a nurse, 2.2 for those without one.

All patients were asked whether they thought it was an advantage or a disadvantage from the patient's point of view when the doctor had a nurse working at the surgery. The majority, three-quarters, felt it was an advantage, less than one in twenty that it was a disadvantage. They were much more likely to see it as an advantage if their doctor worked at a practice with a nurse. The differences are shown in *Table 50.*

Table 50 Patients' views on the advantages or disadvantages of a nurse at the surgery

Patients regard nurse at surgeries:	*Doctor works in practice:**			*All patients*
	With a nurse	*Without a nurse*	*Uncertain*	
	%	%	%	%
Advantage	93	64	73	76
Disadvantage	1	5	2	3
No difference	4	14	8	9
Uncertain	2	17	17	12
Number of patients (=100%)	289	362	163	815

* Based on statements by the patient.

It was the existence of the nurse at the surgery rather than any direct contact with her that seemed to convince people of the advantages, since those who had not had any contact with an existing nurse in the last twelve months were just as likely to see her as an advantage.

The presence or absence of a nurse at the surgery had apparently little effect on patients' view of their doctor. The one significant difference that we have identified is that patients more often thought their doctor had a well equipped up-to-date surgery if a nurse worked there and were more critical of the doctor on this count if he or she did not have one. The proportion describing their doctor as 'not so good' about this was 13% in practices with a nurse, 23% in practices without one. This assessment, as we showed earlier in this section, is a realistic one. The data also suggest that patients may be more likely to consult their general practitioner if they cut their leg and it needs stitching when there is a nurse at the surgery. Among patients who said there was a nurse at the surgery 24% said they would consult their general practitioner in this event rather than go straight to hospital compared with 18% among those who did not think there was a nurse – a suggestive but not quite significant difference. But patients did not think their doctor was better at examining them thoroughly if he worked with a nurse, and the presence of a nurse at the surgery did not affect the likelihood of a patient being examined.* Nor did patients find their doctor any more or less easy to talk to, or any better or worse at explaining things if the primary care team included a nurse at the surgery.

Social workers

Twenty-three per cent of the general practitioners said there was a social worker attached to their practice. The other study with a comparable figure was done in 1969 and found 3% of doctors reporting such an attachment (Irvine and Jefferys 1971). This represents a great rise and although there is no doubt that this type of association has increased, it is possible that the phrase 'attachment' may be interpreted differently. Some doctors may describe an association as an attachment when social services departments would regard it as a liaison. Another study reported that rather over half the local authorities have 'organized links' with general practitioners (Gilchrist *et al.* 1978). In all our twenty study areas at least one doctor reported an attachment whereas one might have expected a few areas not to have any if they were making the same definition as the social services departments. In our 1977 study half, 51%, of the general practitioners who said they did not have a social worker attached to their practice (or 39% of all general practitioners) said they would like to have one attached. So from the doctors' viewpoint, the attachment of a social worker is a frequently desired change in their organization.

Which doctors have them? Attachment of a social worker was unrelated to the number of doctors in a practice: 26% of single-handed doctors had one, compared with 22% of those in a partnership. This is an insignificant difference, although it may be recalled that those working in a health centre were much more likely to have one than other doctors, 38% against 18%, and there were relatively few single-handed doctors in health centres. The reason for these rather strange associations seems to be that older doctors were much more likely to have a social worker attached to their

* 'During the last twelve months, when you've seen a GP, have you had to undress at all, apart from outdoor clothing – so that he could examine you?'

practice than younger doctors: 53% of those aged 60 or more had one compared with 19% of younger doctors. Why should this be so? Does their seniority give them an advantage over their colleagues in obtaining someone in short supply for whom there is a high demand? This seems to be the most probable explanation for what is a surprising finding and a dramatic difference. The figures are in *Table 51.*

Table 51 Doctors' age and the attachment of a social worker

	Doctors' age				*All doctors*
	Under 40	*40–49*	*50–59*	*60 or more*	
	%	%	%	%	%
Social worker attached to practice	24	17	18	53	23
No social worker attached but would like one	42	46	38	19	39
Social worker neither attached nor wanted	34	37	44	28	38
Number of doctors (=100%)	71	120	117	43	357
*Proportion of those without one who wanted one**	56% (54)	55% (100)	46% (96)	40% (20)	51% (275)

* Figures in brackets are numbers on which percentages based (=100%).

How is the attachment of a social worker related to the doctors' attitudes? Doctors with a social worker attached to their practice were no more or less likely to enjoy their work, nor were they any more or less likely to regard it as appropriate for people to seek help from their general practitioners for problems in their family lives. But doctors with a social worker estimated that a relatively *high* proportion of their surgery consultations were for reasons they felt to be trivial, unnecessary, or inappropriate, 38%, compared with the 31% estimated by doctors who did not have a social worker attached. The difference remained if older doctors were excluded.

Among those without a social worker there was no difference between those who wanted one and those who did not, so it does not seem as if doctors who regard a comparatively high proportion of their consultations as trivial, unnecessary, or inappropriate want a social worker to help them to cope with such consultations. Rather it would seem that having got a social worker they may feel that such consultations should be diverted to him or her. On this evidence the social worker does not appear to be making doctors more tolerant or understanding.

However, the attachment of a social worker seemed to do something to improve communications with social services departments – or at any rate the doctors' perceptions of these. Goldberg and Neill (1972) in their study of a social work attachment to general practice also found that 'One of the tangible results . . . is the much easier and more frequent interchange between the general practitioners and the many social services in the area' (p. 172). But the attachment of a social worker did not by any means always solve the problems. Even in practices with a social worker attached a fifth of the doctors regarded communications with social services as poor and only just over a third described them as good. The figures are in *Table 52*.

Table 52 Communications with social services and the attachment of a social worker

	In practices:		*All doctors*
	With social worker attached	*Without social worker attached*	
Doctor regards communications with social services as:	%	%	%
Good	37	20	24
Fair	43	45	44
Poor	20	35	32
Number of doctors (= 100%)	81	274	362

If social workers are making little impact on doctors' attitudes and feelings about their work, are they having any influence on the way doctors communicate with their patients? Contact with a social worker and with the tenets of social work might make doctors more willing to listen to what their patients say or better at explaining things to them. Our data did not suggest that this had happened. That patients with doctors who had a social worker attached to their practice were no more or less likely than others to say they thought they might consult their doctor about a personal problem that was not strictly a medical one can be interpreted in different ways. It might be expected that in practices with a social worker patients would think of going to the social worker in these circumstances rather than to the doctor, and this might make them *less* likely to approach their doctors with such problems. But in fact few patients seemed aware that there was a social worker attached to these practices. Eight per cent of patients whose doctor said there was a social worker attached to his or her practice realized this, and 6% of patients thought there was one when the doctor said there was not! In practices with a social worker rather more patients said they did not know if there was one or not, 71%, compared with 61% of patients in practices with no social worker attached.

Only three patients in the study, less than 0.5%, said they had had any contact with a social worker from the practice during the twelve months before the interview. In a study of a health centre covering over 20,000 patients with a social work attachment scheme the general practitioners referred 216 patients to the social workers in 1977 – a rate of around 1% (Williams and Clare 1979). This suggests that the low contact rate reported on our study may be realistic and not the result of patients' forgetfulness or unwillingness to report such contacts. How aware are they of other members of the practice team?

Table 53 shows that the majority of patients are unaware of the existence of attached staff. A nurse working at the surgery makes an impact on the highest proportion of patients, a social worker attached to the practice the least. Patients feel they would recognize or be aware of a nurse since more said 'no' than 'don't know' about a nurse at the surgery but for the other attachments they were more likely to say they did not know. This seems reasonable given the specialized nature of the work of social workers, health visitors, and midwives.

Table 53 Patients' knowledge of members of the general practice team

	Doctor reported:							
	Nurse at surgery		*Attached social worker*		*Attached health visitor*		*Attached midwife*	
	Yes	*No*	*Yes*	*No*	*Yes*	*No*	*Yes*	*No*
Patient reports people working from the surgery:	%	%	%	%	%	%	%	%
Yes	42	4	8	6	22	2	19	5
No	38	80	21	33	26	30	27	28
Don't know	20	16	71	61	52	68	54	67
Number of patients (= 100%)	455	85	124	406	471	59	426	104

Trainees and medical students

Vocational training schemes and the placement of medical students in general practice have developed alongside the increasing emphasis on team care, and students and trainees are yet other types of people who may be encountered when patients go to visit their doctor. In 1977 three-tenths of the doctors said that their practice took medical students on a regular basis and a quarter said they had trainees.*

Older doctors, aged 60 or more, were less likely to have either students or trainees than younger doctors, while members of the Royal College of General Practitioners were more likely to have them. Few doctors who trained in Asia had medical students in their practice on a regular basis. These differences are shown in *Table 54*. And earlier (*Table 12*) we showed that both students and trainees are more likely to be encountered in practices with four or more doctors than in smaller partnerships.

Associated with these differences, doctors with students or trainees were likely to carry out rather more procedures (their

* 'Do you/does your practice have any trainees – and do you take medical students in the practice on a regular basis: Trainees ——— Medical Students ——— Both ——— Neither ——— ?'

Table 54 Doctors with trainees and medical students

	Proportion with:		*Number of doctors (= 100%)*
	Medical students	*Trainees*	
Date of birth			
Before 1917	12%	10%	42
1917 or later	31%	28%	316
Membership of Royal College of General Practitioners			
Yes	45%	38%	69
No	26%	24%	289
Country of qualification			
Great Britain	33%	28%	295
Northern Ireland or Eire	26%	26%	27
Asia	4%	17%	23
All doctors	30%	26%	362

procedure score was 6.1 compared with 5.3 for other doctors), more of them thought it was appropriate for patients to consult them about problems in their family lives (73% against 63%), and they estimated that a somewhat lower proportion of their consultations were for reasons that were trivial, inappropriate, or unnecessary, 29% compared with 36% on average.

The relationships between having medical students or trainees in the practice and various characteristics and attitudes of the doctor can of course be interpreted in different ways. It is likely that younger doctors and members of the Royal College of General Practitioners are relatively likely to seek and to obtain such placements, but it is also possible that the presence of potentially critical colleagues will stimulate changes both in practices and attitudes.

What were patients' reactions to trainees and to medical students? We did not ask them to distinguish between the two because we felt it would be difficult for them to do so, but in practice trainees are probably more likely to be confused with partners or other deputies for the doctor. Seven per cent of patients said that their doctor had

had a student or trainee with them on at least one occasion when they had consulted him or her. When asked how they did or would feel about students being in the surgery with the doctor 67% said they would not mind in the least, 18% said they would feel a little uneasy, 11% said they would prefer it if the trainee or student left, and 4% made other comments. These proportions were similar for those who had and for those who had not got any experience of a student or trainee sitting in. So unlike those with experience of a nurse or of a receptionist asking them what they wanted to see the doctor about, experience had not made them more or less tolerant and accepting of the presence of a student or trainee. And while two-thirds said they did not mind, the fact that a third had some doubts or substantial reservations indicates that the practice should not be regarded as generally acceptable.

Some comments from those who had had a student or trainee sitting in are given below. First from those who had not minded:

> 'Everybody's got to learn their business. It's the only way they can learn.'

> 'It didn't bother me. I've got past caring now. They've got to learn. You haven't got to object unless you're peculiar.'

Then from those who had felt a little uneasy:

> 'I didn't mind because it was a very small thing but if it was gynaecological I wouldn't like it at all I don't think.'

> 'I'd like to be warned, but I was asked if I'd mind.'

And from those who would have preferred the student or trainee to leave:

> 'The doctor told me who he was and asked if I minded. I know they have to learn. I went with my leg and had a job taking my stocking off and he (the medical student) just sat on the bed and watched me and never helped, just stared and put me off. I was struggling and somebody was watching so that's put me off students.'

> 'Well it was an embarrassing situation. I had an infection in a private place and it was a girl student so I felt embarrassed.'

This last comment was from a man but in general men were much

Table 55 Doctors' perceptions of the advantages and disadvantages of medical students and trainees to patients and to doctors

	Medical students				*Trainees*			
	Doctors with medical students		*Doctors without medical students*		*Doctors with trainees*		*Doctors without trainees*	
	to patients	*to doctors*	*to patients*	*to doctors*	*to patients*	*to doctors*	*to patients*	*to doctors*
	%	%	%	%	%	%	%	%
Advantage	36	70	17	40	59	90	22	52
Mixed feelings	32	17	19	23	32	8	38	24
Disadvantage	14	9	28	15	5	—	17	8
Uncertain	18	4	36	22	4	2	23	16
Number of doctors (=100%)	104	105	222	223	92	92	238	242

more likely to accept medical students or trainees than women, 79% compared with 56% – possibly because the majority of medical students and trainees are men. The difference with age was less marked: if anything young patients were less likely than older ones to accept a student or trainee without question, 62% of those under 35 would do so, 69% of older patients. There was no trend with social class.

More doctors felt that trainees and medical students were an advantage to doctors than thought they were an advantage to patients. And trainees were more often seen as an advantage than medical students to both doctors and patients. Finally doctors with experience of either students or trainees were more likely to see them as an advantage than doctors without such experience. The figures are in *Table 55.*

So while many patients recognize that training on the job may be a good thing in the long run, the immediate experience is not always welcomed and nearly a quarter of the doctors felt that having medical students in the practice was a disadvantage to patients, a similar proportion saw it as an advantage, just over half had mixed feelings or were uncertain.

Other attachments

The attachments considered in this chapter have been the more common ones involving work at the surgery. The position about other types of attachment is shown in *Table 56.* The majority of doctors had both a health visitor and a midwife attached to their practice. In 1969 Irvine and Jefferys (1971) reported that 35% had a health visitor and 26% a midwife employed or attached to their practice. We showed earlier that the majority of patients were unaware of such attachments when they were reported by the doctor but rather more reported some contact with a health visitor, 4%, a midwife, 2%, than with a social worker (less than 0.5%). The attachment of other types of workers such as physiotherapists, psychiatric social workers, chiropodists, dieticians, or marriage guidance counsellors were rare and there was little demand for them from the doctors.

Table 56 Existing and wanted attachments

	Existing	*Wanted**
	%	%
Health visitors	88	9
Midwives	80	5
Social workers	23	39
Nurses seeing patients entirely outside the surgery	51	11
Physiotherapists	1	3
Psychiatric social workers	—	2
Chiropodists	1	1
Dieticians	—	1
Marriage guidance counsellors	1	—
Others	4	3
None	5	52
Number of doctors (=100%)	357	

* 'Would you like to have such people attached, or any more attached?'

In conclusion

The number of people working at doctors' surgeries has risen markedly since 1964. Figures supplied by the Department of Health and Social Security show that between 1966 and 1977 the numbers of secretaries and receptionists (whole-time equivalents) directly employed by a general practitioner increased two-and-a-half times while the number of nurses (again whole-time equivalents) rose seven-fold. Patients are also likely to encounter other sorts of people. But while most patients (around nine-tenths) by 1977 had had some contact with a receptionist, relatively few had received personal care from another professional in the primary care team besides the doctor. One in seven of the patients who had consulted a doctor in a year had been given some help or care by a nurse at the surgery, and the proportion reporting any contact with a social worker was less than one in 100.

The picture of the receptionist as the dragon at the gate was not generally borne out. The majority of patients found the receptionist helpful. But there seemed to be a germ of truth in that concept when they asked patients why they wanted to see the doctor. This provoked some anxiety and antagonism and seemed to discourage some patients from consulting their doctor.

In contrast the presence of a nurse at the surgery if anything increased consultation rates possibly because patients saw the scope of the doctor's work as being wider when he or she worked with a nurse. Although the nurse may have reduced hospital referral for some conditions, these may have been 'replaced' by others which might otherwise have been untreated.

There was little evidence that nurses made any impact on the doctors' attitudes or on the relationship between patient and doctor, but some suggestion that a social worker at the practice had if anything a deleterious effect, since doctors working in practices with a social worker attached regarded a relatively high proportion of their consultations as trivial, inappropriate, or unnecessary. However, it may be that some doctors were mistaken about the existence of formal attachments, and those who identified one may have expected such an arrangement to reduce their level of 'trivia'. When these expectations were not realized they were disappointed and possibly more intolerant. The main advantage of the social worker that we have identified is an improvement in the relationship between general practitioners and social services.

6 General practitioners and hospitals: relationships and roles

What changes have there been in the relationship between general practitioners and hospitals between our two surveys? Has the increase in partnerships, in health centres, in ancillary staff and in equipment at the surgery led to more community rather than hospital care, with patients looking more to general practitioners for help that previously they would have expected to get at the hospital? In this chapter we look first at out-patient attendances at hospital then at patients' attitudes to hospital compared with general practitioner care. Their views of the relative prestige of hospital doctors and of general practitioners leads into a wider discussion of general practitioners' perceptions of their own standing in the community and within the medical profession and to a consideration of the links between general practitioners and hospital, particularly hospital appointments and access to hospital beds.

Attendances at out-patient departments

Contrary to what might be expected from the increase in facilities and staff at general practitioners' surgeries there was a substantial increase in the proportion of patients who said they had attended hospital out-patient or casualty departments in the previous twelve months.* It was 24% in 1964, 36% in 1977. One possible reason for

* 'During the last twelve months have you been to a hospital at all – either as an inpatient or an outpatient or to casualty?'

the increase is a rise in the proportion of people going to hospital for tests and X-rays to which the general practitioner has direct access. And *Table 57* shows that there has been a substantial increase in such facilities.

Table 57 General practitioners' direct access to hospital facilities

	*1963**	*1977*
Skeletal/bone joint X-rays	61%	93%
Barium meal X-rays	47%	78%
Urine micro and culture	85%	97%
Liver function tests	60%	92%
Blood counts	92%	98%
Electrocardiography	8%	58%
Physiotherapy	25%	34%
No. of doctors (= 100%)	141	365

* Cartwright and Marshall (1965).

National statistics for England show that new cases per 1,000 population at *consultant* clinics increased by 2% between 1967 and 1977 (DHSS 1978) so referrals for consultants' advice have not declined either. But while there was little change in the rate of referral to consultant clinics the new case rates at accident and emergency departments rose by 25% between 1967 and 1977. Possibly some patients attending for tests under a direct access scheme were mistakenly included in these figures but the rise is large and suggests that people are going to accident and emergency departments for different reasons and in different circumstances than they had done earlier. Other official figures show the number of attendances per new out-patient at accident and emergency to be falling: from 2.2 in 1959, to 1.8 in 1969, and 1.5 in 1976 (DHSS 1977b).

In 1977 40% of those in the sample who had attended out-patients or casualty reported a single consultation, a further 37% had started attending within the previous twelve months but almost a quarter, 23%, (that is 8% of all our sample) had been going to out-patients for the same condition for a year or more, including 5% of attenders who had been going for five years or longer.

Roughly a quarter of the patients in our sample who had been to hospital out-patients or casualty had gone directly to the casualty department without being referred by their general practitioner. This is the same proportion as in 1964. Seven out of eight of these people who went directly did so after an accident; other complaints they had gone with included violent stomach pains, a burst abscess, pains in the back, a rash that was not clearing up, and a bad nose bleed.

Two out of five of the patients going directly to hospital said it was 'out of surgery hours' or at night, a weekend, or a public holiday. For most of the others the hospital was felt to be more appropriate.

> 'My leg wanted stitching. I knew it was a waste of time going to the doctors because I thought he'd send us to the hospital.'

> 'I've had experience of hospital with this (foreign body in my eye) before and they deal with it quicker and have all sorts of facilities.'

> 'I knew very well he'd send me to the hospital anyway. And I've more confidence going there than going to my own GP. It's an accident hospital and I think they know more than he does.'

One in eight of those going directly said that hospital attention was necessary, some because they needed an ambulance or an X-ray, others because it was 'serious'. One in five felt they needed immediate attention, they could not wait for the doctor, or it was quicker to get to the hospital. One in ten reckoned that hospital attention was better either because it was more specialized, quicker, or better facilities were available, or because they were critical of their general practitioner.

> 'We weren't happy with what the doctor did. He gave me some tablets to take, but the rash got worse.'

All those who had been to out-patients or casualty in the previous twelve months were asked if they felt it was necessary for them to go to hospital or whether they thought a general practitioner could have given them the treatment and tests they had at the hospital. Eighty per cent thought it was necessary to go to hospital, 18% that they could have had the treatment and tests in general practice, and 2% made other comments. Corresponding proportions in 1964 were 83%, 9%, and 8%, indicating an increase in the proportion who felt they need not have gone to hospital. In 1977 the proportion who thought the general practitioner could have treated them was 12%

among those who were referred and 29% among those who went directly to casualty. Comments from some of those who felt they had been referred unnecessarily suggest that a nurse at the surgery might have avoided some of these referrals.

> 'If the GP had a nurse the stitches (taking them out) could have been done at the surgery.'

> 'I think it was a menial task for a doctor' (A course of antibiotics and dressings).

Attendance at a hospital for antenatal care was also felt to be unnecessary by some women.

> 'I had it all first with my GP and then I went to hospital and had it all again. The only difference was I saw the dietician and waited three hours.'

> 'My own doctors were doing the antenatal clinics at the hospital so it seemed stupid to have to drag me right up to hospital when they could have done it at the surgery.'

All the patients who had consulted a general practitioner at all in the previous twelve months were asked if there was any occasion when they felt the general practitioner might have examined them more fully; 11% said yes. This proportion was higher among those who had been to out-patients than among those who had not, 16% compared with 8%. And patients who had been to out-patients were less likely to feel their doctor had a well-equipped, up-to-date surgery: 23% of them described their doctor as 'not so good' about this compared with 15% of those who had not been to out-patients.

At the same time, as in 1964, there was no indication that attendance at out-patients weakened ties between patients and their general practitioners. Patients who had been to out-patients were no less likely to describe their relationship with their doctor as friendly and they were, if anything, rather more likely to say they might consult their doctor about a personal problem; 33% against 25% of non-attenders. A final question to which patients who had been to a hospital out-patient department in the previous year responded differently from those who had not done so asked whether they ever worried that they might waste the doctor's time. Overall 39% said they did or had been concerned about this and the proportion was greater, 46%, among the hospital out-patient or casualty attenders, than among the others, 35%. Possibly anxiety about wasting their own doctor's time causes them to go straight to the hospital.

Turning to the doctors, whether or not patients had been to out-patients or casualty was unrelated to the procedures the doctors carried out, the number of patients they looked after, the number of doctors they worked with, whether a nurse worked at the surgery, their qualifications, use of deputizing services, or their training. These are similar to the results in 1964. But on the more recent study doctors who had a peak flow meter or vitallograph, those who had a microscope, and those who had direct access to physiotherapy had a lower proportion of patients attending out-patient departments. The proportions were 33% when there was a peak flow meter at the surgery, 46% when there was not; 30% when there was a microscope, 40% when there was not, and 29% when the doctor had direct access to physiotherapy, 39% when the doctor did not have this access. There was no difference with the other items of equipment or facilities that were asked about.

Doctors who had access to beds were less likely than others to have patients attending out-patient or casualty departments, 31% against 40%. But this difference seemed to arise because a low proportion of people in rural, that is very low density areas (of less than one elector per hectare in the constituency*) had been to outpatients or casualty, 29% compared with 38% of people in other areas. When density is held constant, the difference between doctors with and without access to beds is smaller and no longer significant.

So once again we have been unable to identify many characteristics of general practitioners which relate to the out-patient consultation rate among their patients. This is not surprising since there are probably conflicting effects: 'active' doctors are likely to send their patients to hospital for tests to which they have direct access, 'inactive' ones to refer them for a consultant's opinion. But the data from patients suggest that some out-patient or casualty attendances would be unnecessary if general practitioners were felt to be more available, were prepared to arrange for more procedures and examinations to be carried out at the surgery and if they could spend more time with some patients. At the same time, 4% of the patients who had consulted their general practitioner in the last twelve months were critical of him or her for *not* sending them to hospital on some occasion. Increasing use of out-patient or casualty depart-

* See Appendix I.

ments may be partly explained by changes in expectations and views about what a general practitioner is likely to do in certain situations and about what it is appropriate for him or her to do. This is considered next.

Patients' attitudes and expectations about hospital and general practitioner care

Patients who had gone directly to a casualty department in the previous twelve months were more likely to expect a general practitioner to send them to hospital with a sprained ankle than were other patients who had been referred to hospital or had not been to hospital as an out-patient at all. The proportions were 41% for those who had gone directly to casualty, 21% of other patients. The proportion who expected to be sent to hospital with a sprained ankle had doubled between 1964 and 1977. And minor surgical procedures were increasingly seen as the province of the hospital. The evidence for this assertion is in *Table 58,* which compares expectations in 1964 and 1977 about whether general practitioners would cope with certain conditions at the surgery or send the patient to hospital.

The proportion who expected referral for a sprained ankle or for the surgical procedures associated with a cyst or abscess had increased. In contrast patients in 1977 were more likely to think the general practitioner would carry out a blood test, and women patients more often expected their doctor to do a vaginal examination in the surgery. This last response may be affected by the increased involvement of general practitioners in family planning.

In the more recent study patients were asked what they would do if they fell at home during the day and thought they had broken an arm. Twenty-four per cent said they would call a general practitioner, 12% would call an ambulance but 59% would go straight to hospital, and 5% thought they would do something else.

People were also asked whether if they cut their leg while at home so that it needed stitching they would be more likely to go to their own doctor or straight to hospital. The proportion who said they would go straight to hospital had increased from 59% in 1964 to 76% in 1977. Only a fifth of patients in the more recent study suggested they would be more likely to go to a general practitioner compared with a third in 1964.

Table 58 Patients' expectations about general practitioners' action or referral for certain conditions

	A sprained ankle		*A small cyst which needed cutting out*		*An abscess which needed opening*		*A blood test*		*A vaginal examination*	
	1964	*1977*	*1964*	*1977*	*1964*	*1977*	*1964*	*1977*	*1964*	*1977*
Patient would expect:	%	%	%	%	%	%	%	%	%	%
General practitioner to cope with it him/herself	81	74	46	42	67	58	56	65	66	79
General practitioner to send them to hospital	12	23	37	51	20	34	30	32	18	14
Uncertain	7	3	17	7	13	8	14	3	16	7
No. of patients (= 100%)	1,326	805	1,332	817	1,329	818	1,328	820	696*	415*

* Women only.

In general the trends in patients' expectations and predicted actions are similar to the trends in doctors' reported actions shown in *Table 59*. In 1977 doctors were less likely to say they stitched cuts 'more often than not', more likely to say they did a vaginal examination with a speculum, and there was no change in their reported actions over excising simple cysts.

Table 59 Changes in general practitioners' reported actions

	Excise simple cysts		*Stitch cuts*		*Do vaginal examination with a speculum*	
	1964	*1977*	*1964*	*1977*	*1964*	*1977*
General practitioner would carry out procedure:	%	%	%	%	%	%
More often than not	29	29	60	44	60	83
Occasionally	33	37	34	43	28	15
Never	38	34	6	13	12	2
Number of doctors (= 100%)	421	362	421	362	421	362

In both 1964 and 1977 patients were asked some questions aimed at establishing their preference for a more hospital or a more general practitioner oriented service. The first related to their preference for a general practitioner who does a number of tests and investigations him or herself or one who sends patients to hospital if they need any investigation. *Table 60* shows that on both occasions the majority preference was for a general practitioner who did a number of tests him or herself and the main difference between the two studies was a decline in the proportion not making an outright choice. Once again patients seem more willing to voice their preferences and expectations in the more recent study.

Patients were then asked: 'If you did not have a general practitioner, but if there was anything the matter with you, you could go straight to the appropriate specialist – how would you feel about that?' After expressing their views they were asked to sum up and say which they would prefer – to have a general practitioner as at present or to go straight to a specialist. Over this the preference, for a general practitioner-based service, was even more clear-cut but

Table 60 Patients' preferences for general practitioner or hospital care

	1964	*1977*
	%	%
Prefers:		
A GP who does a number of tests & investigations himself	50	56
One who sends you to hospital if you need any investigation	35	40
Other comment	15	4
	%	%
Prefers:		
A GP as at present	79	71
To go straight to a specialist	13	17
Specialist a good idea but prefers GP	5	10
Other comment	3	2
Number of patients (=100%)	1,319	816

there was a small increase in the proportion who said they would prefer to go straight to a specialist. This proportion was not affected by recent experience of out-patients or casualty but a higher proportion of those who had been to out-patients than of those without such experience said they would prefer a general practitioner who referred them to hospital if they needed any investigation, 46% compared with 36%.

Some quotations show the main reasons for preferring the general practitioner.

> 'I think I'd rather go to a GP. They seem more down to earth and friendly. I don't think I'd like it (going straight to specialist) very much. The word specialist seems off-putting.'

> 'That (going straight to specialist) supposes you would have a knowledge of health matters and what is wrong with you. You could end up going to see the wrong specialist.'

> 'I don't like that. My GP knows me.'

A number of comments indicate that patients often seem to regard it as more important to save the specialist's time rather than the general practitioner's.

'Yes it would be all right (going straight to the specialist). It might save time often. But you may get people going to a specialist for nothing. I think you've got to have a middle man to say if you should go. You may get specialists crowded out with people with imaginary illnesses.'

'That's going to be very costly to the nation. Everybody will think his sickness is worth taking to the specialist.'

'From a selfish point of view it would be great. But from a practical commonsense point of view it could be a terrible waste of a professional man's time.'

How, then, do they view the relative prestige of hospital specialists and general practitioners?

Doctors' prestige

Most patients think that hospital consultants have more prestige or standing in the community than general practitioners. They also rank both doctors as having a higher prestige than the members of the other professions we asked about. This can be seen from *Table 61*, which also shows that there was remarkably little change in the rankings between 1964 and 1977.

While relative prestige in relation to the six occupations we asked about had not changed, twice as many patients thought that general

Table 61 Patients' ranking of the prestige of six occupations

	*Average rank**	
	1964	*1977*
A hospital specialist (consultant)	1.6	1.6
A general practitioner	2.4	2.6
A headmaster of a grammar school	3.6	3.8
A university professor of history	3.8	3.7
A solicitor who is a senior partner in a small firm	4.0	3.7
A manager of a branch of Marks & Spencer	5.7	5.7
Number of patients making assessments	1,301	771

* 1 = high, 6 = low.

practitioners' prestige had gone down in the community in the last ten years as thought it had gone up. The main explanations they gave for a decline in prestige were first that general practitioners had too many patients, were over-worked or under too much pressure. Some saw this as leading to a deterioration in the doctor-patient relationship.

> 'I think they've got too many patients on their books. They haven't the personal touch any more. I would say that the average person now, unless he is really ill, he'd rather not go to his doctor. They don't seem bothered with you now, you're just another body to them.'

Eleven per cent of all the patients made comments of this sort, while 8% referred to the falling standards of medical care.

> 'They were interested in their work and people's general outlook. I've come to the conclusion that people today aren't really interested in what they are doing but how much money they'll get. That's the tragedy of things today.'

A fall in the doctor's prestige was not always seen as a bad thing.

> 'They've come closer to the people and it's a good thing really. It's made them more approachable.'

> 'I think maybe there's more professionalism in the world today. In the old days a doctor used to stand out. People still need him more than the others.'

Table 62 General practitioners' prestige in the community

	Doctors' views	*Patients' views*
In the last ten years thought prestige of general practitioners in the community had gone:	%	%
Up	3	15
Down	62	33
Not changed	35	47
Don't know	—	5
No. of doctors or patients (=100%)	353	825

Another 4% made comments which could be interpreted as relating to the demystification of medicine.

'I think some of the mysticism has gone out of the profession and the public knows this. People generally are more likely to question the doctor's decision. They accept less the concept of the all-powerful.'

Among the doctors themselves few thought their prestige in the community had risen, the majority thought it had gone down (see *Table 62)*.

The most common reason doctors gave for their fall in prestige was that patients were using and abusing the service more often. A third of the doctors who thought their prestige had declined said this.

'It's decreased because patients now regard the doctor as an employee of the state, to be used if and when they think fit.'

A quarter mentioned changes in the societal view of statuses, concepts of equality, and the general loss of prestige by traditional groups.

'It's decreased due to general aggressive attitudes to any authority.'

Seventeen per cent related their fall in prestige to a decline in their pay and living standards, either relatively or absolutely.

'Decreased because the standard of living has dropped. The gap between the general practitioner and the factory workers and miners is getting closer and closer.'

Fourteen per cent ascribed it to falling standards of care and public conflicts over remuneration.

'It's decreased because of the use of deputizing services, industrial action threats, along with remuneration disputes.'

Thirteen per cent blamed criticism of medicine and the NHS from the media or other outside influences, and 7% thought the dissemination of medical knowledge had contributed to their fall in prestige.

There was some consensus between patients and doctors that general practitioner's prestige in the community had fallen, but at the same time a third of the doctors thought that *within the medical profession* the prestige of the general practitioner had gone up in the last ten years, one in eight that it had gone down, and just over half that it had not changed.

Over a third of the doctors who thought their prestige in the profession had risen suggested that the recognition of the importance of primary care was a reason. Twenty-nine per cent mentioned improved standards in general practice, 21% that there was now more contact between general practitioners and hospitals, and 17%

Table 63 Doctors' views on increased prestige of general practitioners within the medical profession by various characteristics and circumstances

	Proportion thinking relative prestige of general practitioners within the medical profession had risen in the last ten years	*No. of doctors (=100%)*
Partnership		
Yes	36%	303
No – single handed	19%	43
Date of birth		
Before 1917	20%	44
1917 or later	35%	300
Hospital appointment		
Yes	42%	140
No	28%	209
Access to hospital beds		
Yes	43%	152
No	26%	198
Member of Royal College of General Practitioners		
Yes	57%	69
No	28%	277
Trainer		
Yes	68%	31
No	30%	315
Believes patients more knowledgeable		
Yes	38%	250
No	24%	98

that more was now done in general practitioners' surgeries. A belief that their prestige in the medical profession has increased may be an index of morale and if this is so morale was relatively low among single-handed doctors and older doctors born before 1917 (see *Table 63*). There was no trend with the size of partnership or among other age groups. Nor was morale related to working in a health centre. It was high among those who were members of the Royal College of General Practitioners, among trainers, and among those who thought patients were more knowledgeable now.

Doctors who thought their prestige in the medical profession had risen were also more likely to think that relationships between general practitioners and hospitals had improved; 44% of them did compared with 23% of other doctors. Altogether 30% of doctors felt relationships had improved, and 28% that they had deteriorated. Nearly three-quarters of the doctors who thought relationships were better mentioned more contact with the hospital, and better communication. One doctor commented:

> 'Improved because of mixing of GPs and consultants at regular postgraduate meetings.'

Among doctors who felt relationships with the hospital had deteriorated nearly a third mentioned increasing hospital waiting lists and falling standards of care, a similar proportion that contact with consultants and hospital staff was less, and a quarter suggested that lowered morale of hospital staff had contributed.

Forty-two per cent of members of the Royal College of General Practitioners compared with 27% of non-members, and 44% of trainers compared with 26% of others thought relationships with the hospital were better. In these respects doctors who thought relationships had improved were similar to those who felt their prestige in the medical profession had risen. Surprisingly, only 18% of doctors born since 1937 but 33% of older doctors thought relationships had improved, and doctors' views on this were not associated with either hospital appointments or access to hospital beds. Hospital connections are considered next.

Hospital links

The proportion of general practitioners with a hospital appointment had risen markedly from 23% in 1964 to 40% in 1977. This rise was counterbalanced by a decrease from 36% to 24% in the proportion wanting an appointment, leaving the proportion who neither had one nor wanted one roughly similar. Possibly the increase in partnerships and partnership sizes has enabled more general practitioners who wanted one to take on such appointments. Only a third of those in partnerships of three or less had an appointment compared with half of those in larger partnerships. At the same time hospital authorities have probably looked more to general practitioners to help them with their service needs. Unfortunately we do not have any data on the specialties in which general practitioners were working.

In contrast access to hospital beds where they retained full responsibility for their patients had not increased significantly in the period between the two studies: it was 39% in 1964, 43% in 1977.* And this too was related to the number of doctors they worked with, rising from a quarter of single-handed doctors to half of those in partnerships of four or more. But the proportion who wanted beds – or more beds – had fallen from 72% in 1964 to 61% in 1977. In both studies the proportion among those with beds who wanted more was higher than the proportion among those without any beds who wanted some (84% and 66% respectively in 1964, 72% and 54% in 1977).

General practitioners who had hospital appointments in 1977 were more likely to have access to beds than those without such an appointment, 56% compared with 34%. Two-fifths of all doctors had neither, just over a fifth had both. Not surprisingly, with this overlap, doctors with the two different types of hospital link shared similar characteristics (see *Table 64*). They were relatively young, and better qualified than those without such links. In addition those with hospital appointments were more likely to be members of the Royal College of General Practitioners. Doctors were also more likely to have a hospital appointment if they looked after a relatively small number of patients. The proportion with one was 53% of those who looked after less than 2,000 patients and fell to 29% of those with 3,000 or more. There was no such trend in the proportion with access to hospital beds.

Obviously distance from the hospital may be important but our

* 'Do you, as a general practitioner, have direct access to any NHS beds where you retain full responsibility for treatment of your patients whilst in hospital?'

Table 64 Variations in hospital appointments and access to hospital beds with various characteristics of the doctor

	Proportion of doctors with:		*Number of doctors (=100%)*
	A hospital appointment	*Access to hospital beds*	
Doctor's date of birth			
Before 1917	11%	29%	44
1917–26	38%	44%	118
1927–36	47%	45%	121
1937 or later	51%	48%	73
Qualifications			
Licentiate only	17%	27%	41
Degree only	36%	40%	190
Further qualification	54%	53%	128
Member of Royal College of General Practitioners			
Yes	54%	49%	70
No	37%	42%	289
Time it normally takes to get from surgery to nearest hospital with a casualty department			
Less than 5 mins.	48%	52%	102
5< 15	38%	41%	162
15< 30	38%	29%	76
30 minutes or longer	25%	60%	20
Area density			
Very low	52%	69%	77
Low	41%	38%	90
Medium low	34%	26%	73
Medium high	38%	50%	52
High	31%	51%	39
Very high	34%	9%	32
All doctors	40	43	363

only data relate to the time it took doctors to get to the nearest hospital with a casualty department and in rural areas particularly doctors may have access to beds in hospitals without such a department. But there was some indication that those with a hospital appointment had surgeries a relatively short distance away from a hospital with a casualty department. Doctors in very low density areas were the ones most likely to have access to beds, while few of those in very high density areas (with 50 or more electors per hectare) had one.

Table 65 Some variations in practices between doctors with and those without hospital appointments or hospital beds

	Hospital appointment		*Access to beds*		*All doctors*
	Yes	*No*	*Yes*	*No*	
	%	%	%	%	%
*Nurses in the practice**					
Attached	70	65	79	60	67
Employed	44	30	39	34	35
Neither	8	21	6	23	16
Average number of nights a week on call	2.2	2.3	2.4	2.1	2.3
Uses deputizing service	%	%	%	%	%
Regularly	23	28	21	30	26
Occasionally	13	22	12	23	18
Never	64	50	67	47	56
Regards consultation between themselves and hospital medical staff over discharge of patients as adequate	%	%	%	%	%
Yes	29	35	29	35	32
No	71	65	71	65	68
Practice has:					
ECG machine	52%	32%	53%	30%	40%
Haemoglobinometer	40%	33%	40%	33%	36%
Peak flow meter or vitallograph	88%	71%	88%	70%	77%
Microscope	53%	42%	51%	43%	46%
Refrigerator	94%	93%	97%	91%	94%
Average procedure score	6.0	5.4	6.1	5.3	5.6
Number of doctors (=100%)	141	216	154	203	358

* These percentages add to more than 100 as some practices had both an attached and an employed nurse.

Doctors with either type of hospital link had direct access to a greater number of hospital facilities than those without such connections. Of the seven facilities asked about (skeletal X-rays, barium meal X-rays, urine micro and culture, liver function tests, blood counts, electrocardiography, and physiotherapy) those with hospital appointments had access to 5.8 on average, those without to 5.3 and the comparable figures for those with and without access to beds were 6.0 and 5.1. Some other variations in their practices are shown in *Table 65.*

Doctors with either type of hospital connection more often had a nurse working at the surgery: more of those with hospital appointments employed a nurse, those with access to beds more often had an attached nurse. Working at a hospital in either capacity did not mean that they were less often on call at night but they were *less* likely to use a deputizing service. Having a hospital appointment or access to beds did not make them any less critical of the consultation with hospital medical staff over discharge of patients. Those with hospital links worked in practices that had rather more equipment and they were more likely to carry out certain procedures themselves. Did this mean that they put more emphasis on clinical procedures and possibly less on the social, community, and family aspects of their work?

In fact doctors with hospital links were no more or less likely to regard it as appropriate for people to seek help from their general practitioners for problems in their family lives, and those with access to beds regarded a rather *lower* proportion of their surgery consultations as trivial, inappropriate, or unnecessary – an estimated average of 29% compared with 36% for those without access. A similar difference was also found in 1964. A relatively low proportion of those with a hospital appointment regarded it as very important for different members of a family to go to the same doctor: 20% compared with 30% of those without an appointment. Having a hospital appointment or access to hospital beds did not appear to affect the importance they attached to continuity of care nor the emphasis they would like to see on community care or a team approach in the future.

Again, as in 1964, a comparatively small proportion of those with access to beds said they enjoyed their work 'not very much' or 'not at all': 5% compared with 11% of those without such access, and in 1977 there was a similar difference for those with and those without hospital appointments (also 5% and 11% respectively). This time we also asked doctors about their conditions of work under the NHS. The proportions who described themselves as being very or fairly happy with them were 66% of those with access to beds, 56% of those without. There was no difference between those with and those without hospital appointments.

Did their patients perceive any difference between doctors with or without hospital links? A comparison of patients whose doctor has a hospital appointment with those whose doctor did not have one showed that more middle-class than working-class patients had doctors with such a link: 46% compared with 34%. There was no difference for doctors with hospital beds. This time, in contrast to the findings in 1964, we found middle-class patients no more critical than working-class ones so class variations did not appear to contribute to different levels of criticisms of doctors with and without hospital appointments. In practice, our findings in 1977 were that patients of doctors with hospital appointments were less likely than others to be critical of their doctors about visiting (5% compared with 12%), taking time and not hurrying them (11% compared with 18%), listening to what they say (3% compared with 9%), and explaining things (14% compared with 26%). There were no differences in the number of consultations or home visits reported by the two groups of patients, nor in their assessment of their relationship as being friendly or businesslike. Neither were there any differences in their overall satisfaction with their care, or whether they knew their doctor well. They were no more or less critical of their doctors about examining them and they were as likely to say they would consult over a personal problem that was not strictly medical.

Patients were less critical of their doctor for not explaining things fully when their doctor had access to hospital beds than when he or she did not: 17% against 25% described their doctor as 'not so good' about this.

Clearly many of the characteristics of the doctors with hospital links are interrelated – their age, qualifications, size of partnership, practice facilities, and attitudes to their work and consultations. The differences we have observed may be either effects or causes of their hospital ties. Both the differences and the lack of differences are noteworthy; the differences because they suggest certain trends and clusterings, the lack of differences because they indicate an absence of what might be seen as possible undesirable side effects of a hospital connection. The clustering relates hospital connections with younger, better qualified doctors, working in larger groups with more facilities, and performing a wider range of clinical tasks. This was not accompanied by a restriction in their perceptions of their social role and in some ways their relationships with their patients seemed rather better than colleagues without such links.

Discussion

Again the changes or lack of changes between 1964 and 1977 are disappointing. In spite of the increases in partnerships, in ancillary staff, and in facilities at surgeries, more patients are going directly to hospital accident and emergency departments when they have small accidents which need immediate attention. Morgan *et al.* (1974) found 78% of the patients attending accident and emergency departments in Newcastle upon Tyne were 'self-referred' and they identify self-referral as one of the major problems facing the accident and emergency services. The accessibility of hospital care 'being open 24 hours a day' and weekends was an important factor as it was on the present study in which over a quarter of the self-referred patients assessed that a general practitioner could have done what the hospital did.

While minor surgical procedures are increasingly seen as the province of the hospital there was some indication that by 1977 the general practitioner was expected to do more investigations. But the increase in direct access to facilities did not appear to have had much effect on patients' expectations nor on referral rates for consultant advice.

Horder (1977) believes: 'A new relationship is emerging between two sorts of doctors (specialist and generalist) with different and complementary functions, but on the same level.' He contrasts this with the past when general practitioners 'considered the relationship was in some respects as superior to inferior, with functions that were often the same.' Our data suggest some movement in this direction with a third of the general practitioners believing that their prestige in the medical profession had risen in the past ten years. In contrast their prestige in the community was thought by both patients and doctors to have fallen rather than risen, but this appeared to be part of a general decline in professional prestige. Within the professions both consultants and general practitioners retained their pre-eminence.

Armstrong (1979) also argues that in the period between our two surveys the perceived power of the hospital within the medical community has been declining. Both he and Horder imply a decline in general practitioners' desire for hospital work and hospital beds that was not substantiated by our findings.

7 Variations between doctors

In earlier chapters some variations between doctors of different ages and doctors with different types of qualifications have been mentioned. Here the variations are brought together and further ones explored. The chapter starts with basic characteristics of sex and age, then moves on to look at the country in which the doctors qualified, their vocational training since qualification, and membership of the Royal College of General Practitioners. Finally their list sizes and the types of areas in which they work are considered.

Sex

The proportion of women doctors in our 1964 sample was 5%; by 1977 this had doubled. Another difference was that in the earlier study three-quarters of the women doctors' patients were women whereas in the more recent study it had dropped to three-fifths and did not differ significantly from the 51% for men doctors. In 1977 the women doctors had rather younger patients than their male colleagues: the proportion under 55 was 62% for men, 75% for women doctors. And related to this, patients had been with their female doctors for a shorter time: 14% of them had been with the doctor for fifteen years or more compared with 32% of those with male doctors. However, there were no significant differences between men and women *doctors* in the length of time they had been in their present practice nor in their dates of birth.

In general it is the *lack* of difference between men and women general practitioners which is most notable. They did not differ in their qualifications, number of partners, whether or not they had a nurse working at the surgery or in the importance they attached to continuity of care and family care. Nor did they differ in the emphasis they would like to see on team care, community care, or home visiting. Similar proportions thought it was appropriate for people to seek help from their general practitioner with problems in their family lives and they estimated similar proportions of their consultations as being trivial, unnecessary, or inappropriate.

Main differences were that women doctors had rather fewer patients; 49% of them estimated that they looked after 2,500 patients or more compared with 69% of male doctors. But more women doctors said they sometimes used a deputizing service, 70% against 41%; and they were on call for fewer nights on average, 1.7 compared with 2.3 in a week. Rather surprisingly women were less likely to say they fitted IUDs 'more often than not' when the procedure arose in their practice, 16% of them said this, 31% of the men; and although more women said they would examine vagina with a specula 'more often than not', 92% against 83%, this difference might have occurred by chance. On our overall procedure score men had a higher average, 5.7, than women, 4.8.

As far as their patients were concerned the two groups reported similar consultation rates and similar numbers of home visits. There was no difference in their general satisfaction with their care but patients of women doctors were more likely to describe their doctor as 'not so good' about taking time and not hurrying them: 24% of them made this criticism, 13% of patients with a male doctor. This was a criticism made more often by patients under 55 but even when the comparison is confined to patients under 55 the difference still persists, 31% of those with a woman doctor made the criticism, 17% of those with a man. Patients were no more or less likely to regard women doctors as being good at listening to them or explaining things or as being 'good with children'. Neither did they differ in their description of their relationship as 'friendly' or 'businesslike'. But the women who had a female doctor were *less* likely to say they might consult their doctor about a personal problem that was not a strictly medical one, than women who had a male doctor, 15% compared with 32%. There was no difference between male patients with male and female doctors and no overall difference between men and women patients over this.

So there is no evidence that women general practitioners are adopting a more expressive role than their male colleagues. How far this lack of difference stems from the selection process – deciding to take up a career in which men predominate and being accepted by that profession – or in the socialization process of the medical school and the medical profession, it is impossible to say. But as the proportion of women doctors increases more differences in attitudes and practices may emerge.

Age

In earlier chapters we showed that older doctors were less likely to have hospital appointments or access to hospital beds. They were more often single-handed or in small partnerships of two doctors.

Table 66 Variations in practices with doctor's date of birth

	Date of birth				*All doctors*
	Before 1917	*1917–26*	*1927–36*	*1937 or later*	
Practice has an:					
ECG machine	16%	36%	36%	64%	40%
Peak flow meter or vitallograph	63%	74%	83%	83%	77%
Haemoglobinometer	40%	42%	33%	28%	36%
Uses deputizing service:	%	%	%	%	%
Regularly	38	26	26	19	26
Occasionally	23	19	21	10	18
Never	39	55	53	71	56
Has appointment system for:	%	%	%	%	%
All surgery consultations*	52	74	70	68	69
Some surgery consultations	25	16	20	21	19
None	23	10	10	11	12
Number of doctors (= 100%)	44	119	120	72	362

* Except emergencies.

And they less often had a nurse working at the surgery. Some other differences in their practices are shown in *Table 66*.

Younger doctors more often worked in practices with an ECG machine or a peak flow meter but it was the older doctors who were more likely to have a haemoglobinometer. There was no difference in their average procedure score. Older doctors more often used a deputizing service but less often had an appointment system for all their surgery consultations. It seems likely that the latter variation is a generation effect while the former may be a genuine 'effect' of age and smaller partnerships as doctors may well become less willing to turn out at night as they get older.

Some ways in which their attitudes varied are shown in *Table 67*.

Table 67 Variations in doctors' attitudes with their date of birth

	Date of birth				*All doctors*
	Before 1917	*1917–26*	*1927–36*	*1937 or later*	
Family care felt to be:	%	%	%	%	%
Very important	43	27	25	17	26
Fairly important	39	48	46	58	49
Relatively unimportant	18	25	29	25	25
In future development would like to see:	%	%	%	%	%
More emphasis on community care	49	55	64	76	62
Less emphasis	14	9	12	3	9
No change	37	36	24	21	29
More emphasis on	%	%	%	%	%
health education	71	72	82	83	78
Less emphasis	7	8	5	3	6
No change	22	20	13	14	16
Feels appropriate patient to see GP about family problem	65%	75%	63%	61%	67%
Number of doctors (= 100%)	43	116	119	71	357

Older doctors attached more importance to family care but did not differ from their younger colleagues in the importance they attached to continuity of care, nor in the emphasis they would like to see in the future on home visiting and team care. However the older doctors were somewhat less enthusiastic than younger ones about

Table 68 Doctors' date of birth and length of time in practice, length of time patients had had their doctor and how well patients knew their doctor

	Doctor's date of birth				*All doctors*
	Before 1917	*1917–26*	*1927–36*	*1937 or later*	
Length of time doctor had been in particular practice:	%	%	%	%	%
Less than a year	2	1	1	6	2
1 year < 2 years	—	2	1	8	3
2 years < 5 years	5	2	6	37	11
5 years < 10 years	5	3	13	36	13
10 years < 15 years	2	11	36	13	19
15 years < 20 years	19	13	35	—	18
20 years or more	67	68	8	—	34
No. of doctors (= 100%)	42	115	118	70	352
Length of time patient had been with particular doctor:	%	%	%	%	%
Less than a year	9	7	8	19	10
1 year < 2 years	7	5	9	14	9
2 years < 5 years	17	13	15	36	18
5 years < 10 years	12	17	25	19	18
10 years < 15 years	9	16	20	6	15
15 years or more	46	42	23	6	30
How well patient knew doctor:	%	%	%	%	%
Very well indeed	17	25	14	13	18
Reasonably well	37	32	34	24	32
Fairly well	25	23	27	31	26
Not well	18	15	21	24	19
Never consulted that doctor	3	5	4	8	5
No. of patients (= 100%)	112	278	255	145	819

putting more emphasis on health education and definitely less enthusiastic about an increasing emphasis on community care. They did not differ in their estimates of the proportion of surgery consultations which they felt were trivial, unnecessary, or inappropriate, nor in the extent to which they said they enjoyed their work as general practitioners, but, as shown before, it was the doctors in their fifties who were the most likely to feel it was appropriate for people to seek help from their general practitioners for problems in their family lives.

It might have been expected that older doctors would attach more importance to continuity of care since they were likely to have been in the same practice longer than their younger colleagues. In fact general practitioners move from practice to practice remarkably little: seven-tenths of all doctors and nine out of ten of those aged 50 or more had been in the same practice for at least ten years. This can be seen from *Table 68*, which also shows the extent to which the length of time patients had been with their doctor was related to the doctor's age. Naturally patients tended to have been with the older doctors for longer but there was relatively little variation with the doctor's age in the proportion of patients who said they knew their doctor 'very well indeed', although this was clearly related to how

Table 69 Age of doctors and variations in the proportion of patients consulting in different periods

	Doctor's date of birth				*All doctors*
	Before 1917	*1917–26*	*1927–36*	*1937 or later*	
Proportion of patients who had:					
Consulted a general practitioner in the previous twelve months	70%	72%	79%	80%	75%
Consulted a general practitioner in the previous two weeks	6%	11%	15%	16%	12%
Had a home visit from a general practitioner in the previous twelve months	13%	19%	19%	28%	19%
No. of patients (= 100%)	110	275	257	147	825

long they had been with their doctor. (This was shown in *Table 15.*)

In considering the relationship between the doctor's age and patient's views and experiences it is helpful that the age of patients and doctors were not correlated. However the sex of the patients did vary with the doctor's age. Younger doctors have more women patients: the proportion fell from 59% for doctors under 40 to 42% for those aged 60 or more.

Patients of older doctors were less likely to have consulted their doctor in the last twelve months, and the proportion who had consulted a general practitioner in the previous two weeks showed a similar difference as did the proportion reporting a home visit in the previous twelve months. The figures are in *Table 69.*

Other studies (Williams 1970) have reported somewhat similar findings in relation to consultation rates. What is the mechanism? People with older doctors were no more likely to say that they worried about wasting the doctor's time* or that they had put off consulting the doctor because he was too busy.** A possible explanation lies in what Sowerby (1977) has described as a 'ritual of courtship'. Our data suggest that people are more likely to consult their doctor at least once during a year when they have been with him a comparatively short period of time than when they have been with him for longer. The proportion consulting at least once fell from 82% of those who had been with the doctor for less than five years to 75% of those who had been with their doctor for between five and fifteen years and to 67% for those who had been with their doctor for a longer time. It did not vary between those who had been with him for less than a year, between one and two years, and between two and five years, so the high proportion for this group was not just a result of consulting when people had first registered with a doctor. A three-way analysis suggests that it is the length of time patients have been with a doctor rather than the age of the doctor which influences the likelihood of consultations (see *Table 70*).

Patients with older doctors were no more – or less – likely to have been to hospital as an in-patient or out-patient in the last twelve months, and there was no variation with the age of the doctor in the proportion of patients who thought they might discuss a personal problem they were worried about with their doctor.

* 'Do you ever worry that you might waste the doctor's time?'

** 'In the last twelve months have you ever put off consulting the doctor because you felt he was too busy?'

Table 70 Proportion of patients consulting a general practitioner in previous year by age of doctor and length of time they had had their doctor

	Proportion consulting		
	Length of time patient had had doctor		
	Less than 5 years	*5 yrs<15 yrs*	*15 yrs or more*
Doctor's date of birth:			
Before 1917	78% (37)	74% (23)	62% (52)
1917–26	82% (71)	73% (90)	65% (118)
1927 or later	84% (182)	76% (151)	76% (67)

Figures in brackets are numbers on which percentages are based *(=100%).*

In view of the differences in type of practice and in the organization and facilities available, the relative lack of difference as far as the patients were concerned is, in some ways, surprising.

Country of qualification

Earlier, in Chapter 4, we showed that doctors who had trained abroad were more likely to work in health centres than those who trained in Great Britain (England, Wales, and Scotland).

Other variations with country of qualification are shown in *Table 71.* Doctors who qualified in Asia were younger on average than those who qualified in Great Britain, whereas the Irish doctors were older as were those who qualified elsewhere. (Ten of the twelve in this last category qualified in Europe.) In spite of the fact that Irish doctors were generally older they were not more likely to be in single-handed practices. They seemed to have a preference for three-doctor practices. Relatively few doctors who trained in Great Britain said they looked after 3,000 or more patients and they were more likely to work in low density areas. No Asian doctors in our sample worked in the areas of very high density: they clustered in areas of medium density, and they were the ones most likely to work in designated or open areas where there are relatively few general practitioners per head of the population.

Doctors who qualified in Britain were more likely than the others to have access to hospital beds and to have direct access to various

Table 71 Characteristics of doctors who trained in different countries

	Great Britain	*Eire or Northern Ireland*	*Asian*	*Elsewhere*	*All doctors*
Date of birth:	%	%	%	%	%
Before 1917	11	18	—	(59)	12
1917–26	33	52	8	(33)	33
1927–36	34	15	67	(8)	34
1937 or later	22	15	25	(—)	21
Number of doctors works with:	%	%	%	%	%
On own	11	11	17	(33)	13
Two	26	15	21	(41)	25
Three	25	48	33	(—)	26
Four	22	22	21	(8)	22
Five or more	16	4	8	(8)	14
Looks after 3,000 or more patients	35%	59%	45%	(50%)	38%
Area density:	%	%	%	%	%
Very low	25	7	4	—	21
Low	27	11	25	(17)	19
Medium low	17	29	46	(25)	20
Medium high	13	25	25	(8)	14
High	11	14	—	(8)	11
Very high	7	14	—	(42)	15
Type of area:	%	%	%	%	%
Designated	14 } 39	30 } 52	25 } 71	(—) } (42)	16 } 42
Open	25 }	22 }	46 }	(42) }	26 }
Intermediate	43	33	21	(33)	40
Restricted	18	15	8	(25)	18
Member of the Royal College of General Practitioners	22%	14%	0%	(17%)	19%
Access to hospital beds	46%	22%	33%	(33%)	43%
Proportion with direct access to:					
Barium meal X-rays	81%	75%	67%	(33%)	78%
ECG	64%	50%	17%	(42%)	58%
Liver function tests	94%	79%	83%	(92%)	92%
Physiotherapy	37%	21%	13%	(25%)	34%

continued

Table 71 continued

	Great Britain	*Eire or Northern Ireland*	*Asia*	*Elsewhere*	*All doctors*
Qualifications:	%	%	%	%	%
Licentiate only	13	7	—	(8)	12
Degree with or without licentiate but no further qualifications	% 51	% 64	% 58	% (75)	% 54
Some further qualifications	36	29	42	(17)	34
Practice has attached:	%	%	%	%	%
Health visitor	89	93	67	(78)	88
Midwife	81	78	88	(78)	80
Social worker	20	37	38	(44)	23
Nurse working outside surgery	49	56	54	(67)	51
Other person	7	7	—	(—)	6
None	4	4	8	(22)	5
Proportion sometimes using a deputizing service	41%	61%	57%	(75%)	44%
Average procedure score	5.7	5.2	5.3	(5.1)	5.6
Number of doctors (=100%)	285	27	22	10	348

Percentages and averages in brackets are based on less than twenty doctors.

facilities. In addition more of them were members of the Royal College of General Practitioners, but they were no more likely than doctors qualifying elsewhere to have further qualifications.

There were no significant differences between the groups in relation to their sex, whether or not they had a hospital appointment, the proportion of their patients who were elderly (aged 65 or more), or whether they had a nurse working in the surgery. But there were some differences in other sorts of attachment. Asian doctors were relatively unlikely to have a health visitor attached to

Table 72 Variations in doctors' attitudes with country of qualification

	Doctor qualified in:				*All doctors*
	Great Britain	*Northern Ireland or Eire*	*Asia*	*Elsewhere*	
Average proportion of surgery consultations felt to be trivial, inappropriate, or unnecessary	31%	39%	53%	(34%)	33%
Thinks it appropriate for people to seek help from their general practitioner with problems in their family lives	69%	81%	29%	(67%)	67%
Regards it as very important for different members of a family to go to the same doctor	24%	11%	50%	(58%)	26%
In the future would like to see:					
Less emphasis on community care	7%	11%	29%	(25%)	9%
More emphasis on health education	76%	70%	96%	(100%)	78%
More emphasis on team approach	43%	54%	96%	(60%)	49%
Wants access to some, or to more, hospital beds	60%	48%	88%	(67%)	61%
Number of doctors (=100%)	282	26	24	11	349

the practice while those qualifying in Britain were least likely to have a social worker attached. Doctors who qualified in Britain were less likely to use a deputizing service and they carried out rather more procedures themselves; but this last difference arose because more of them worked in very low density or rural areas.

Not surprisingly doctors who qualified in different countries differed in their attitudes to their work in a number of ways (see *Table 72*). The ones who differed most were those who qualified in Asia.

Another study (Smith, D.J. 1980) showed that doctors who qualified overseas (among whom Asians predominated) were more likely than doctors who qualified in Britain to have become general practitioners against their inclination. Related to this Smith also found that the overseas general practitioners had spent longer in the hospital service in Britain than had their British colleagues. This experience may explain their apathy with regard to some aspects of general practice. As *Table 72* shows Asian doctors perceived a relatively high proportion of surgery consultations as being for trivial, inappropriate, or unnecessary reasons and few felt it was appropriate for patients to consult them for problems in their family lives. This contrasts with the emphasis they put on family ties as they were relatively likely to regard it as very important for different members of a family to go to the same doctor. They also tended to want more emphasis on health education and on a team approach, but less emphasis on community, rather than hospital care.

In general, those who qualified in Asia seemed rather more hospital oriented than the others. They were the ones most likely to want access to some, or to more, hospital beds. When asked what they enjoyed about their work as general practitioners 18% of them compared with 7% of other doctors mentioned clinical medicine or treating people with medical problems. And 42% of them against 56% of the others said they enjoyed their work as general practitioners 'very much'. However, these last two differences might have occurred by chance with the small numbers in our sample.

What of their patients? The age distribution of patients was similar for doctors qualifying in different countries but patients with doctors who qualified in Asia had been with the same doctor for a shorter time and associated with this they said they knew their doctor less well. They were also more likely to have consulted a general practitioner in the last twelve months. The data are in *Table 73.*

Table 73 The patients of doctors who qualified in different countries

	Doctor qualified in:				
	Great Britain	*Eire or Northern Ireland*	*Asia*	*Elsewhere*	*All doctors*
How long with same doctor:	%	%	%	%	%
Less than a year	9	6	18	5	10
1 year<2 years	9	4	12	—	9
2 years<5 years	17	18	31	19	18
5 years <10 years	18	21	23	19	18
10 years<15 years	15	15	7	24	15
15 years or more	32	36	9	33	30
Knows own doctor:	%	%	%	%	%
Very well	18	30	10	19	18
Reasonably well	34	22	25	38	32
Fairly well	26	27	25	19	26
Not well	17	17	34	24	19
Never consulted	5	4	6	—	5
Proportion who had consulted a general practitioner in the previous 12 months	75%	78%	85%	57%	75%
Proportion of middle-class patients	45%	30%	32%	40%	43%
No. of patients (=100%)*	625	66	66	21	805

* With a doctor.

Although doctors who qualified in Asia were less likely to regard it as appropriate for patients to consult their general practitioners for problems in their family lives, their patients were no less likely than patients whose doctors qualified in Britain or elsewhere to say they might consult their doctor about a personal problem.

Doctors who qualified in Britain had a higher proportion of middle-class patients than doctors who qualified elsewhere. This might mean that their patients would be rather more critical, but on the other hand, criticism tended to be related to how well patients knew their doctors, which would lead to the expectation that patients of doctors who qualified in Asia would be the most critical. The differences we found are in *Table 74.*

Table 74 Patients' views and doctors' country of qualification

	Doctor qualified in:				*All doctors*
	Great Britain	*Eire or Northern Ireland*	*Asia*	*Else-where*	
Proportion of patients describing doctors as 'not so good' about:					
Having a pleasant, comfortable waiting room	27%	41%	37%	(44%)	29%
Always visiting when asked	8%	17%	13%	(33%)	10%
Sending people to hospital when necessary	5%	10%	11%	(17%)	6%
Keeping people waiting in his/her waiting room	18%	28%	33%	(29%)	20%
Examining people carefully and thoroughly	10%	14%	22%	(22%)	12%
Listening to what you say	5%	10%	16%	(17%)	7%
Explaining things fully	19%	25%	33%	(28%)	22%
Patient feels it is:	%	%	%	%	%
Easy to talk to doctor and ask him/her questions	83	76	67	(55)	80
Not possible to talk as much as you like	16	22	30	(39)	19
Other comment	1	2	3	(6)	1
Patient considers relationship with doctor:	%	%	%	%	%
Friendly	31	43	19	(28)	32
Businesslike	67	54	81	(72)	66
Other comment	2	3	—	—	2

continued

Table 74 continued

	Doctor qualified in:				*All doctors*
	Great Britain	*Eire or Northern Ireland*	*Asia*	*Else-where*	
Last problem consulted doctor for:	%	%	%	%	%
He/she explained adequately	77	75	61	(50)	75
Patient wanted more information	18	15	36	(22)	19
Other comment	5	10	3	(28)	6
Views on own care:	%	%	%	%	%
Very satisfied	52	42	29	(28)	49
Satisfied	40	49	54	(50)	42
Mixed feelings or dissatisfied	8	9	16	(22)	9
Other comment	—	—	1	—	—
Number of patients with a doctor they had consulted (=100%)	563	58	60	17	715

Over a number of issues it was the patients of doctors who qualified in Britain who were the least critical. It was also clear that patients with doctors who qualified in Asia were more critical of their doctors, mainly over communication issues but also over examining. They were also more likely to have reservations when asked a general question about the care they had received from their own doctor. The higher level of criticism about these doctors cannot be dismissed entirely on the grounds that patients are prejudiced, because of the differences we found in the doctors' views and practices.

Training

Doctors were asked whether they had had any specific training for general practice after qualifying. *Table 75* shows the types of training that were listed together with the replies.

Table 75 Specific training for general practice

	All types	*Priority*
	%	%
Recognized vocational training scheme	2 }	26
Trainee year in general practice	25 }	
Self-organized vocational training scheme	15	12
Assistantship in general practice	32	22
Other training	10	4
No specific training	36	36
Number of doctors (=100%)	358	

Several doctors indicated that they had had more than one type of training, but for further analyses they have been classified in one way, taking as our priority the order listed in *Table 75.*

Almost half the doctors under 50 had had a trainee year or some sort of vocational training compared with a quarter of the older doctors. More of the older ones had had an assistantship but half of those aged 60 or more had had no specific training. These differences are shown in *Table 76.* For subsequent analyses we have combined the recognized and self-organized trainee schemes together with those who had a trainee year in general practice.

Table 76 Training and date of birth

	Before 1917		*1917–26*		*1927–36*		*1937 or later*	
	%		%		%		%	
Trainee year or recognized vocational training scheme	5 }	19	18 }	28	41 }	48	28 }	49
Self-organized vocational training scheme	14 }		10 }		7 }		21 }	
Assistantship	29		30		17		12	
Other training	—		3		6		4	
No specific training	52		39		29		35	
Number of doctors (=100%)	44		118		116		75	

Associated with the age difference in assistantships, more single-handed doctors than others had had an assistantship; 35% against 20%, and more of those who qualified in Eire or Northern Ireland had done so: 41% compared with 20%. In addition doctors who had had an assistantship were the least likely to work in a practice with an attached or employed nurse. Altogether 80% of the doctors with any training worked in a practice with a nurse compared with 91% of those without any training. And those with training were not particularly enthusiastic about a team approach in general practice. This can be seen from *Table 77*.

Table 77 Training and employment and attachment of nurses and views on team approach

	Trainee year or vocational training scheme	*Assistantship*	*No specific training*	*All doctors**
Practice has:	%	%	%	%
Attached nurses only	48	47	52	49
Employed nurses only	18	7	20	17
Both	16	22	19	18
Neither	18	24	9	16
Views on future emphasis on team approach in general practice. Would like to see:	%	%	%	%
More emphasis	48	40	52	49
Less emphasis	16	21	11	15
No change	34	39	37	36
Other comment	2	—	—	—
*Number of doctors (=100%)**	133	90	126	355

* Includes the 13 with other types of training.

Overall there was no relationship between having or not having attached or employed nurses and the emphasis doctors placed on a team approach. Possibly a trainee year or an assistantship makes some doctors more self-reliant and less likely to feel the need for a nurse. However, their training was not related to the procedures they carried out themselves.

Members of the Royal College of General Practitioners were more likely to have had a trainee year or a vocational training scheme, 49% of them had done so compared with 35% of non-members. But there were no trends with size of partnership. Nor were there any differences in training associated with working in a health centre, having a group practice allowance, using a deputizing service, or having a hospital appointment.

Training was also unrelated to the extent to which they said they enjoyed general practice or to their estimates of the proportion of consultations that were trivial, unnecessary, or inappropriate. Nor did it relate to their views on whether it was appropriate for people to seek help from their general practitioners for problems in their family lives.

These results are rather surprising and disappointing, particularly when put alongside the attitudes and practices of trainers. As *Table 78* shows trainers* were more likely to feel it was

Table 78 A comparison of trainers and other doctors

	Trainers	*Other general practitioners*
Proportion who:		
Regarded it as appropriate for people to seek help from general practitioners for problems in their family lives	86%	65%
Regarded less than a quarter of their surgery consultations as trivial, inappropriate, or unnecessary	68%	48%
Work in practices with attached or employed nurses	94%	83%
Were members of the Royal College of General Practitioners	39%	18%
Number of doctors (=100%)	29	323

* Based on data about the doctors in our study from the Department of Health and Social Security.

appropriate for people to seek help from their general practitioners for problems in their family lives, they regarded fewer of their consultations as trivial, inappropriate, or unnecessary, and they more often worked in practices with attached or employed nurses. They were no more or less likely to use a deputizing service than other doctors.

In addition trainers were more likely to say they enjoyed general practice very much, 74% of them did so compared with 54% of other doctors. Possibly the trainers get more out of the vocational training schemes than the trainees.

Turning to patients' views of their doctors, it is possible to compare the attitudes of patients who had general practitioners with different types of training. It appears that doctors with a trainee year or a recognized vocational training scheme were more often regarded as easy to talk to by their patients and they were also more often felt to be good about visiting when asked. But these differences

Table 79 Doctors' training and patients' views

	Trainee year or recognized vocational training scheme	*Self-organized vocational training scheme*	*Assistant-ship*	*No specific training*
Patient regarded general practitioner as:				
Easy to talk to and ask questions	89%	77%	74%	79%
Good about visiting when asked	76%	57%	71%	65%
Good about taking time and not hurrying them	86%	87%	76%	84%
Good about having a well-equipped, up-to-date surgery	79%	84%	66%	78%
No. of patients (= 100%)	130	69	90	167

did not apply to doctors with a self-organized vocational training scheme so are difficult to interpret. Those who had had an assistantship were least often felt to be good at taking time and not hurrying them and at having a well-equipped, up-to-date surgery (see *Table 79*). There were no significant differences in patients' general satisfactions with their own care, in their views about whether the doctor was good about explaining things to them or examining them thoroughly. And patients did not rate trainers any more or less highly than other doctors in these respects.

The main impact of vocational training schemes may be in the future. But results here give little cause for complacency. Our conclusions may be contrasted with those of Freeman and Byrne (1973, 1976, and 1977) which seem to be accepted as demonstrating the value of such schemes (Horder 1977). Freeman and Byrne showed improvements in 'clinical factual recall' and 'problem-solving skill in patient management'. They did not look at any patients' assessments and although they looked at trainees' attitudes the results of those assessments have not yet been published.

Membership of the Royal College of General Practitioners

A fifth of the doctors who completed our questionnaire were members of the College. The proportion did not vary with the doctor's age, but as we have just seen College members were more likely to have had a trainee year or a vocational training scheme.

Members and non-members differed little in their types of practice: they had similar numbers of partners and list sizes, they carried out similar numbers of procedures, and similar proportions worked in practices with attached and with employed nurses. But as we showed earlier (*Table 64)* College members were more likely to have hospital appointments; they were also less likely to use a deputizing service (32% against 47%). And as shown in *Table 54* they were more likely to work in practices taking trainees and medical students on a regular basis.

The two groups differed more in their attitudes. College members were more likely to feel that the prestige of general practitioners within the medical profession had gone up in the last ten years, and that relationships with the hospital had improved. They were also less likely to feel that their prestige in the community had gone

Table 80 Attitudes of members of the Royal College of General Practitioners

	Member	*Non-member*
Proportion believing:		
Relative prestige of general practitioners in the medical profession had gone up in the past 10 years	57%	28%
Relationships between general practitioners and hospitals had improved	42%	27%
General practitioners' prestige or standing in the community had gone down	49%	66%
It is appropriate for people to seek help from their general practitioners for problems in their family lives	76%	65%
Estimated average proportion of surgery consultations felt to be trivial, inappropriate, or unnecessary	22%	36%
Number of doctors (=100%)	68	277

down. They were possibly more likely to feel that it was appropriate for patients to seek help from their general practitioners with problems in their family lives, and they estimated that a lower proportion of their consultations were for reasons they felt to be trivial, inappropriate, or unnecessary. These results are in *Table 80*. But they did not differ in the importance they attached to family care or to continuity of care nor in the emphasis they would like to see on team care.

It might be expected from the observed differences that College members would be more likely to say they enjoyed their work as general practitioners but, as in 1964, there was no difference between College members and others over this.

Of course we cannot tell how far the differences in attitudes existed before they became members. It is possible that some of these views stimulated them to join the College. And having joined, the atmosphere and contacts at the College might well foster a sense that the prestige and influence of their professional group was increasing. It is perhaps sad that this does not appear to add to their enjoyment of their work. Possibly some doctors join the College because they are dissatisfied with some aspects of their job.

Patients did not find doctors who were members of the Royal College of General Practitioners any better or worse at explaining things, being easy to talk to, listening to what they said, taking time, and not hurrying them. Nor were they any more or less critical of their doctors about examining them or being prepared to visit when asked.

List sizes

Doctors were asked to estimate the approximate number of NHS patients that they themselves looked after.* This distribution is compared in *Table 81* with the average size of list from DHSS data. For partnerships these are based on the total number of patients divided by the number of partners. The doctors' estimates are higher probably because of the way the sample was chosen. A doctor's chance of being included was related to the number of patients he or she looked after, so the average within a partnership is likely to be lower than that for the doctors identified by the patients. The doctors' estimates of the number of patients they look after have been taken in the following analyses.

Table 81 Estimates of list sizes

	Doctors' estimates	*DHSS estimates*
Number of NHS patients:	%	%
Less than 1,500	2	5
1,500–1,999	8	16
2,000–2,499	23	32
2,500–2,999	29	28
3,000 or more	38	19
Number of doctors (= 100%)	346	354

As there is no retiring age in general practice this could be a profession from which people retire gradually, either reducing the number of patients on their list if they are single-handed or taking responsibility for a smaller proportion of the practice work if they

* 'What is the approximate number of patients on your list? If in partnership, please estimate the number of NHS patients that you yourself look after (to the nearest 100).'

are in partnership. But this does not seem to happen. The only clear difference with age in 1977 as in 1964 was that a relatively small proportion of younger doctors, aged 40 or less, looked after 3,000 or more patients: 24% of them compared with 42% of older doctors.

Doctors' estimates of the numbers of patients they personally looked after were not related to the number of partners they worked with nor to whether they worked in a practice with a treatment room. More surprisingly doctors looking after a relatively large number of patients were no more or less likely to be in practices with either an employed or an attached nurse working at the surgery. This suggests that nurses are not being used to enable doctors to look after more patients. On the other hand, among those working with a nurse at the surgery, the nurse was more likely to stitch cuts if the doctors looked after a lot of patients. The proportions doing so rose from 7% if the doctor looked after less than 2,000 patients to 26% of those looking after 3,000 or more. The number of procedures the doctors carried out themselves did not vary with the number of patients they looked after. And those with large and small list sizes were as likely to have medical students or trainees at the practice. Ways in which their practice organization did differ were that doctors looking after larger numbers of patients were more likely to have appointment systems for all their surgery consultations; this proportion rose from 56% for those looking after less than 2,000 to 72% for those with 3,000 or more (see also Bridgstock 1976). And those with larger lists were also more likely to make use of deputizing services (the proportion doing so rose from 38% to 60%).

As far as their attitudes were concerned, the extent to which doctors said they enjoyed their work was unrelated to the number of patients they looked after, so too were their views on the appropriateness of general practitioner consultations for personal problems. But the proportion of surgery consultations that they felt were for trivial, unnecessary, or inappropriate reasons rose from 24% of those looking after less than 2,000 patients to 38% of those looking after 3,000 or more. At the same time, when they were asked what proportion, if any, of their consultations they would like to be able to spend more time on, the average rose from a third to a half. But the proportion who went on to say they would like to spend more time with patients with psychiatric or emotional problems *fell* from 62% of those with less than 2,000 patients to 41% of those with 3,000 or more.

There was no evidence from the patients that the care they got from their doctors varied with the number of patients the doctors looked after. Consultation rates, home visit rates, and patients' assessment of their care and of their relationship with their doctor were similar whether the doctor looked after relatively small or large numbers of patients. Doctors with small lists were more likely to have hospital appointments, the proportion fell from 53% of those looking after less than 2,000 patients to 29% of those who said they looked after 3,000 or more. Those doctors with appointments at any rate may not have more time to spend with the patients in their practice.

The most noteworthy difference that we have identified is that those with larger lists regard more of their consultations as 'trivial'. There is also some evidence that they are less interested in emotional and psychiatric problems. In 1964 we observed a tendency for the proportion of patients consulting their doctor in the previous twelve months to decrease as the doctor's size of list increased. One speculation about the possible reason for this difference was that some patients, particularly people who were mentally disturbed, sought out doctors who were sympathetic to their problems and prepared to spend time and listen to them. Our 1977 data provide some support for this explanation but none for the initial difference!

One other variation with list size was the type of area the doctors worked in (see Appendix I) and some area variations are examined next.

Types of areas

To what extent does Hart's (1971) inverse care law, 'the availability of good medical care tends to vary inversely with the need of the population served', operate within general practice? Can we pinpoint any differences between doctors in better and less well off areas? And are there major differences between urban and rural areas? Finally, what of the efforts of the DHSS to encourage a more equitable distribution of doctors?

In looking at these questions we have taken three classifications. One is by politics. Nine of the twenty study constituencies returned a Labour Member of Parliament in October 1974, eleven a Conservative one. This is clearly related to patients' social class. In the Labour areas 30% of the patients in our sample were classified as middle-class whereas the proportion in the Conservative areas was 54%. Another is by density, that is the number of electors per hectare. This ranged from under one in the relatively rural constituencies of Workington, Stratford on Avon, West Derbyshire, and Monmouth, to over 50 in Lambeth Streatham and the City of Westminster, Paddington (see Appendix I). The third division is by whether the DHSS have classified the doctor as working in a 'designated area', that is an area with a low ratio of doctors to patients where the Department offers a financial inducement to try to attract more doctors, 'an open area' where there are no inducements or restrictions, or 'intermediate or restricted areas' where there are different levels of restrictions on new doctors moving into the area.

The three classifications are related. Seven of the nine Labour areas were designated or open while nine of the eleven Conservative ones were intermediate or restricted. Seven of the nine low density areas were Conservative, five of the seven high density ones were Labour. Seven of the nine low density areas were intermediate or restricted, three of the seven high density ones.

Politics

Doctors in Labour constituencies had larger lists than those in in Conservative areas. They did not differ in the number of partners they worked with nor in their dates of birth but more of those in Conservative areas had had a trainee year in general practice or a recognized vocational training scheme, while more of those in Labour areas had trained in Asia, 12% compared with 2%. Those in Conservative areas had more links with the hospital: they were more likely to have hospital appointments and direct access to various facilities, but no more likely to have direct access to hospital beds. The doctors in Labour areas did not compensate for this lack of access by carrying out more procedures themselves nor by having more equipment. Rather the reverse. And they were also less likely to have the stimulation of trainees and medical students. There were no differences between the two groups in the proportion with nurses working at the surgery nor in other attached staff. But more of the doctors in Labour areas used a deputizing service.

Turning to their attitudes, doctors working in Labour constituencies were rather more likely to think it was inappropriate for patients to consult them about problems in their family lives and they felt

Table 82 Doctors in Labour and Conservative areas

	Lobour area	*Conservative area*
Proportion:		
Looking after 3,000 or more patients	51%	28%
With trainee year or vocational training scheme	21%	31%
With hospital appointment	32%	46%
With direct access to		
Skeletal X-rays	88%	97%
Barium meal X-rays	64%	88%
Liver function tests	88%	94%
ECG	52%	63%
Physiotherapy	22%	43%
Average procedure score	4.9	6.1
Proportion:		
Using deputizing service	62%	31%
In practice taking trainees	21%	31%
In practice taking medical students	19%	37%
In practice with refrigerator	90%	96%
In practice with an ECG machine	31%	47%
In practice with a microscope	38%	53%
Thinking it inappropriate for patients to consult about problems in family lives	32%	23%
Enjoying work in general practice 'very much'	50%	60%
Believing general practitioners' prestige in the medical profession had gone up	25%	40%
Very or fairly happy about their conditions of work under the NHS	51%	68%
Average proportion of consultations felt to be trivial, unnecessary, or inappropriate	36%	30%
Number of doctors (=100%)	150	196

that a higher proportion of their consultations were for trivial, inappropriate, or unnecessary reasons. They were less likely to feel happy about their conditions of work under the NHS and less likely to feel that general practitioner prestige had risen in the medical profession.

These differences are shown in *Table 82.* Together they indicate that the Labour constituencies are rather more deprived in relation to primary health care than Conservative ones. This is further evidence to support Hart's inverse care law since politics are related to social class and the General Household Survey (1977) has shown a clear association between chronic ill health and socio-economic group.

Density

Contrary to some expectations the proportion of single-handed doctors increased with density, rising from 9% in the very low density areas to 25% in the very high density areas. Related to this doctors in the high density areas tended to be older: 19% of them were 60 or more compared with 9% in the low ones. Few doctors in the very low density areas compared with those in other areas looked after 3,000 or more patients (18% against 43%), but more of them had hospital appointments (52% against 37%) and access to beds (69% compared with 36%). No doctors in the very high density areas worked in health centres compared with 24% in other areas. This proportion was also relatively low at the opposite end of the scale. Few doctors in the low or very low density areas used a deputizing service. The doctors in the very low density areas also carried out more procedures themselves, their score was 6.7 against 5.3 for the others. They also had more equipment. As for direct access to various hospital facilities the groups that stood out were the doctors in the high density areas as being less likely to have direct access to either skeletal or barium meal X-rays while few of those in medium-low density areas also had direct access to barium meal X-rays or to ECGs. The distribution of all these characteristics for which differences have been found are shown for the six density groups in *Table 83.* There were no marked differences in their vocational training nor in membership of the Royal College of General Practitioners.

As far as their attitudes were concerned, doctors in very low density areas made the lowest estimate of the proportion of surgery

Table 83 Doctors in areas of varying density

	Density – no. of electors per hectare					
	Under 1 very low	*1<5 low*	*5<20 medium low*	*20<30 medium high*	*30<50 high*	*50+ very high*
Proportion:						
Single-handed	9%	11%	12%	10%	15%	25%
Aged 60 or more	9%	10%	8%	16%	26%	16%
Looking after 3,000 or more patients	18%	34%	45%	54%	42%	48%
With hospital appointments	52%	41%	34%	38%	31%	34%
With access to hospital beds	69%	38%	26%	50%	51%	9%
Working in health centres	14%	31%	26%	21%	26%	0%
Using a deputizing service	12%	13%	56%	77%	85%	81%
With ECG machine at practice	59%	44%	22%	35%	36%	38%
With peak flow meter or vitallo-graph	86%	73%	77%	77%	69%	78%
With direct access to skeletal X-rays	100%	96%	92%	96%	69%	94%
With direct access to barium meal X-rays	91%	87%	53%	90%	59%	78%
With direct access to ECGs	71%	57%	27%	62%	79%	72%
Average procedure score	6.7	5.9	5.1	5.4	4.6	4.6
Average proportion of 'trivial' consultations	27%	34%	34%	35%	31%	40%
Number of doctors (=100%)	74	89	71	48	36	29

consultations that they felt to be trivial, inappropriate, or unnecessary, but there were no differences in the proportions believing it was appropriate to be consulted about problems in peoples' family lives, nor in the proportions who said they enjoyed their work 'very much'.

For the patients, it was perhaps surprising that there were no differences in the time they estimated it took them to get to the doctor's surgery but the way they got there differed markedly; the proportion going by private transport dropping from 58% in the very low density areas to 13% in the very high ones, while the proportions who walked all the way were 31% and 69% at the two extremes.

The low density areas contained a relatively high proportion of middle-class patients, 48% against 39% in all the other areas combined, but the proportion was highest of all in the very high density areas, 61%. Possibly in the big cities it is the middle-class ones who get on to the electoral register (see Smith, C. 1981). There was no relationship between density and either the length of time people had had the same doctor or in consultation or home visit rates. But people in the very low density areas were less likely to have been to hospital out-patient departments in the previous twelve months; 29% of them had done so, 38% of those in other areas. They were more likely to say they were very satisfied with their own medical care, 58% against 47%; and more of them regarded their doctor as easy to talk to, 86% compared with 79%.

To sum up the findings on density, our results indicate fairly large differences between the ways doctors practice in different areas, some but not all of these relating to density, and they suggest doctors in country or very low density areas give a rather wider service to their patients.

Designated and other areas

The variations in list size between these types of areas are given in *Table 84*. This shows that for large lists the doctors' estimates of the number of patients they looked after was more directly related to the type of area than the DHSS estimates. But for small lists it is the reverse.

The proportion of patients living in designated areas (where the DHSS is trying to encourage more doctors) was similar in 1964 and 1977, 16% and 18% respectively, but the proportion in intermediate

Table 84 Type of area and size of list

	Type of Area			
	Designa-ted	*Open*	*Intermediate*	*Restricted*
Doctors' estimates of number of patients looked after:	%	%	%	%
Less than 2,000	4	9	10	18
2,000–2,499	9	22	24	33
2,500–2,999	21	32	36	20
3,000 or more	66	37	30	29
List size (from DHSS data):*	%	%	%	%
Less than 2,000	7	13	24	41
2,000–2,499	25	37	32	27
2,500–2,999	14	38	30	21
3,000 or more	54	12	14	11
Number of doctors (=100%)	56	91	133	61

* For doctors working in partnerships this is the average list size of the partnership.

and restricted areas had increased markedly from 8% to 52%, indicating a much greater use of restrictive policies at the later date. And whereas in 1964 a relatively high proportion of younger doctors were working in designated areas – presumably attracted by the Ministry's incentives – this was not so in 1977. Unpublished figures from the DHSS for 1978 also show no difference in the age distribution of doctors working in designated areas and other areas. And only 8% of the doctors in designated areas had been in the same practice for less than five years against 16% in other areas – an insignificant difference but in the direction which indicates that current policy is not attracting new doctors to the undoctored areas. The problem is that the designated and open areas are less attractive to doctors: 49% of the doctors in those areas said they enjoyed their work very much compared with 60% of those in both restricted and intermediate areas.

8 Some variations in patients' attitudes and care

In this chapter we discuss differences between men and women, between people of different ages, and between those in different social classes. But age is related to both sex and social class. Women live longer than men: in our sample 51% of people aged 18–64 were male, but only 38% of people aged 65 and over. In addition older people were more likely than younger ones to be classified as working-class: 63% of those aged 55 and over were classified as working-class, but only 54% of younger people. The association between age and social class probably reflects a decrease over time in the proportion of men in jobs classified as working class (see Reid 1977). Because of these associations our discussion of consultation rates and how they have changed over time considers the inter-relationships with patient's sex, age, and social class.

Sex, age, social class, and consulting the doctor

Most studies report higher consultation rates for women than for men (Verbrugge 1979) – ours is no exception. In 1977 80% of women but only 71% of men reported some consultation with their doctor (or his partners, assistant, or locum) in the previous 12 months, and 9% of men compared with 5% of women said they had not consulted a general practitioner in the previous five years. The figures for consultation by age and sex are in *Table 85.* These show that the main difference between men and women is that women consult more often than men during the reproductive ages. Among

Table 85 Age, sex, and frequency of consultation with general practitioner

	Men							
	18–24	*25–34*	*35–44*	*45–54*	*55–64*	*65–74*	*75+*	*All ages*
Number of consultations in previous twelve months:	%	%	%	%	%	%	%	%
None	27	31	26	38	28	29	14	29
One	20	26	23	15	12	17	14	19
2–4	33	26	33	25	27	27	34	29
5–9	11	12	12	12	15	5	19	12
10 or more	9	5	6	10	18	22	19	11
Estimated average	3.0	2.5	2.8	3.0	4.1	4.0	4.8	3.2
Number of men (=100%)	45	81	78	67	67	41	21	400

	Women							
	18–24	*25–34*	*35–44*	*45–54*	*55–64*	*65–74*	*75+*	*All ages*
Number of consultations in previous twelve months:	%	%	%	%	%	%	%	%
None	9	12	19	29	16	31	33	20
One	7	17	20	19	25	15	2	16
2–4	28	42	34	32	32	22	29	32
5–9	32	14	10	13	9	25	19	17
10 or more	24	15	17	7	18	7	17	15
Estimated average	6.1	4.3	4.0	2.8	4.0	3.4	4.2	4.0
Number of women (=100%)	46	85	59	62	68	60	42	425

those aged 18–44, women reported an average of 4.6 consultations in the previous year compared with an average of 2.7 for men.

Because of the higher consultation rate for younger women the pattern of consultations by age was different for men and women. Among men the 55–64 age group marks a clear increase in the consultation rate. Men aged 55 and over consulted more frequently than younger men – this was not because more of the older men consulted at all, but because those who consulted did so more frequently. For women the consultation rate was relatively high among those aged 18–44, presumably because of attendances for family planning and for antenatal services. The rate was lowest for women in the 45–54 age group–women who are often regarded as having relatively high consultation rates because of problems associated with the menopause. However, women in this age group generally no longer need to consult for reasons associated with childbearing and are probably not yet experiencing the problems associated with old age. Data from the General Household Survey 1977 support this finding. They show a relatively low rate among women aged 45–64; an average of 3.9 compared with 4.3 for women aged 15–44 and 4.2 for those aged 65–74.

On the whole, the patterns of consultation by age and sex in our data and from the General Household Survey are in good agreement, except that the General Household Survey reports higher consultation rates than us for women aged 65 or more and men aged 75 or over. The figures are given later in *Table 87*. This adds to our suspicion that our rates are unduly low for these older age groups, particularly the older women.

Turning to social class differences we found that similar proportions of people classified as working-class and middle-class had consulted the doctor in the previous 12 months, but working-class people had a slightly higher annual consultation rate, an estimated 4.0 compared with 3.3 for middle-class people. The figures are in *Table 86*, which shows that these social class differences exist only among the men, not among the women, and that the difference is clear for men aged 18–54 and for older men. (We have divided our sample into these two broad age groups because they show the major differences that we found with age.)

The higher consultation rates of working-class men under 55 probably reflects the higher risks of accidents and chronic illness associated with their employment, as well as their greater need to present sickness certificates. For the older men the higher consultation rate of working-class men may also be due to poorer adjustment by working-class men to retirement – a suggestion which receives some support from the study by Haynes, McMichael, and Tyroler (1977) of mortality after retirement among rubber workers.

It was noted earlier in Chapter 3 that, in comparison with 1964, the estimated overall consultation rate has risen, but not significantly, from 3.4 to 3.6 per person in 1977. However, within age, sex, and social class groups there have been some clear changes. These can be seen in *Table 86.* Men, in 1977, consulted their general practitioners more often than men in 1964, but the increase is entirely due to the higher consultation rate of working-class men in 1977 compared with 1964. One factor that may contribute to this change is that working-class men may be receiving more preventive and screening services now, particularly for hypertension. In 1977 we found no difference between middle- and working-class men in the proportion who said they had had their blood pressure tested in the previous twelve months, but a higher proportion of working- than of middle-class men (20% compared with 13%) said they had never had it tested. There was no difference between middle- and working-class women in either of these two proportions. Another possibility is that the level of sickness for which working-class men consult their doctor has changed. Certainly more working-class men in 1977 said they would consult their general practitioner about 'a constant feeling of depression for three weeks': 78% said they would do so compared with 62% in 1964. But this proportion had also increased for middle-class men and for both middle- and working-class women so this cannot explain why the consultation rate of working-class men has increased markedly in comparison with other groups.

The consultation rates recorded in the General Household Surveys of 1971 and 1977 are presented in *Table 87.* It is clear that in those studies there is a marked fall in the consultation rates of both men and women aged 65 and over. This decline may in part be related to the drop in home visiting. Other factors which may contribute to a decrease in the dependency of older people on general practitioners are the setting up of day hospitals and possibly a decrease in disability as a healthier generation moves into old age and has the benefit of more effective medical treatment.

A final change over time revealed in our analyses by age, sex, and

Table 86 Age, sex, social class, and number of consultations in 1977 and 1964

	1977							
	Men				*Women*			
	18–54		*55+*		*18–54*		*55+*	
	Middle Class	*Working Class*	*Middle Class*	*Working Class*	*Middle Class*	*Working Class*	*Middle Class*	*Working Class*
Number of consultations in last twelve months:	%	%	%	%	%	%	%	%
None	30	30	36	22	20	14	26	26
One	27	17	13	15	13	20	20	14
2–4	27	31	33	24	35	33	25	28
5–9	13	11	8	14	16	17	18	16
10+	3	11	10	25	16	16	11	16
Estimated average	2.3	3.2	3.0	4.9	4.2	4.3	3.6	3.9
No. of people (=100%)	116	151	48	79	114	123	61	103

	1964							
	Men				*Women*			
	21–54		*55+*		*21–54*		*55+*	
	Middle Class	*Working Class*	*Middle Class*	*Working Class*	*Middle Class*	*Working Class*	*Middle Class*	*Working Class*
Number of consultations in last twelve months:	%	%	%	%	%	%	%	%
None	36	40	33	32	30	27	27	33
One	27	19	18	10	18	12	8	8
2–4	27	26	19	31	30	29	28	22
5–9	5	8	12	9	10	15	14	16
10+	5	7	18	18	12	17	23	21
Estimated average	2.1	2.4	3.7	3.9	3.2	4.0	4.6	4.4
No. of people (= 100%)	143	295	74	136	165	249	88	177

Table 87 Average number of consultations per person per year in England and Wales, 1971 and 1977

Age	*Men*		*Women*	
	1971	*1977*	*1971*	*1977*
15–44	2.4	2.4	4.5	4.3
45–64	3.4	3.6	4.2	3.9
65–74	5.0	3.8	5.3	4.2
75+	6.8	6.1	7.4	5.1

Source: General Household Surveys 1971 and 1977.

social class is an increase in the consultation rate between 1964 and 1977 among younger, middle-class women – from 3.2 to 4.2. Again this is probably due to the increased use of the general practitioner for contraceptive services.

Men and women

Apart from the somewhat different ways and rates at which men and women consult their general practitioner are there other differences in their attitudes or experiences?

In 1964 it appeared that women put a somewhat stronger emphasis than men on personal relationships and this, along with their more frequent contact with their doctor, was thought to explain why women seemed more attached to their doctor as a person and less willing to consult partners or locums. In 1977 too women appeared to identify more strongly with their particular general practitioner. Discussing their consultations in the previous twelve months, 80% of women said they had seen their own doctor only or mainly; this was true for only 71% of the men. Women were less prepared to see some other doctor in the practice, only 27% said they would 'not mind in the least' seeing another doctor if theirs was not available, but 41% of men felt this. In addition, when asked whether they would wait half an hour to see their own doctor even though they could see another doctor in the group straight away, 51% of men but 60% of women said they would rather wait. In practice a higher proportion of women said they had waited an hour or more at their last surgery consultation. Eleven per cent of them had done so compared with 5% of men.

About half of both men and women thought that general practitioners worked too many hours a week, but women were more sensitive about wasting the doctor's time. Forty-three per cent of women, compared with 36% of men said they sometimes worried they might waste the doctor's time, and when asked if, in the last twelve months, they had ever put off consulting the doctor because they felt he or she was too busy, 15% of women said they had done so compared with 9% of men. Neither of these findings can be attributed to age variations. Men and women were equally likely to think their doctor was good about taking time and not hurrying them.

When we asked people about the qualities in their general practitioner that they appreciated, women were more likely to mention that the doctor had patience, took time, and did not hurry them, and that the doctor put them at ease – he was approachable. Men more often mentioned the doctor's honest, straightforward approach, and more frequently commented on the quality of the doctor's medical care (see *Table 88*). These results are similar to those from 1964.

Table 88 Sex and some of the qualities appreciated in their general practitioner

	Men	*Women*	*Both sexes*
Qualities appreciated in general practitioner:			
Listens, takes time, doesn't hurry you, has patience	22%	32%	27%
Approachable – 'can take any problem', 'puts you at ease'	21%	30%	26%
Blunt, frank, straightforward, talks 'man to man', honest	11%	7%	9%
Some reference to medical care	65%	55%	60%
Number of people (= 100%)	346	377	723

There was no difference between men and women in the proportion who had been visited at home by their doctor in the previous year, nor in the number of times they had been visited. However 13% of women praised their doctor for visiting promptly, regularly, when asked, or without grumbling compared with 8% of men; and when asked specifically whether they thought their doctor was good or not so good about visiting when asked, 73% of women described the doctor as good, but only 63% of men. Women may be more appreciative of the doctor's willingness to visit because of their experiences with children, but in contrast to 1964 women were no more likely than men to praise the doctor for being good with children in 1977.

Another observation in 1964 was that men had a greater orientation towards the hospital. In 1977 too men appeared more ready to use hospital services. Although there was no difference in the proportions who said they had attended hospital out-patients or casualty in the previous twelve months (34% of men and 38% of women), men were more likely to have taken themselves to the casualty department without being referred by their general practitioner: 39% of men attending out-patients or casualty had gone there directly compared with 18% of women. Nearly all of these patients attended with some problem caused by an accident. Younger people were more likely to have gone direct to casualty, and the sex difference is clear only for people aged 18–44.

We asked whether, if they cut their leg while at home, so that it needed stitching, they would be more likely to go to a general practitioner or straight to the hospital. Women were more likely than men to say they would go to their general practitioner: 27% compared with 15%. Differences in their reasons centred around the issue of time and convenience. Eleven per cent of women, but 4% of men said they would be treated more quickly by the general practitioner, and would get more immediate attention. In contrast, 27% of men compared with 18% of women thought the hospital was more accessible and that they would be treated more quickly there. Differences in relative ease of access did not explain these preferences. A further question in 1977 asked people what they would do if they fell at home during the day and thought they had broken an arm. Men were, again, more likely to say they would go direct to hospital; 66% of them said this compared with 53% of women.

Although men seemed more inclined to use hospital services in 1977 they were no more likely than women to want a system in which they had direct access to specialists. Nor in 1977 did men prefer, more frequently than women, a general practitioner who sent them to hospital for any investigation whereas in 1964 more men than women expressed a preference for going directly to specialists and for a general practitioner who would send them to hospital if they needed any investigation. In this sense the greater hospital orientation of men is less clear than it was in 1964.

'Men seem slightly less conservative and more prepared to think of different types of organisation.' This was one conclusion from the 1964 study and, although as we have just shown there was no longer a difference between men and women in 1977 in the proportion preferring a system in which people could go directly to specialists, there was still some evidence that men were more ready to consider changes and more willing to accept care from another doctor. Twenty per cent of men compared with 15% of women preferred an emergency doctor service rather than arrangements made between their own doctor and other local general practitioners for night calls. This is similar to 1964, when comparable figures were 22% and 12%.

Although men were not in general more critical of their doctors than women, and they were no more or less satisfied with the care they got from their doctor, more men said they had thought of changing their doctor: 12% compared with 7% of women. And rather more men than women thought it would be very or fairly easy to change their doctors: 54% of men thought this, 46% of women.

More men than women, 33% compared with 26%, said they would like to have a private doctor if they could afford it rather than keep an NHS one.* But there were no differences in the proportions wanting to change to or from an appointment system or preferring a single-handed doctor rather than one who worked in a partnership. Their views on the advantages and disadvantages of a nurse working in the surgery were similar. There was no difference in the proportion of men or women who would, on some occasions, prefer to see a doctor of a particular sex. A quarter of the men said they would like to see a male doctor sometimes, and 21% of the women specified a female doctor on occasion. In 1964, 29% of women said there were occasions when they would prefer to see a woman general practitioner rather than a man. Possibly the more direct way in which the question was worded affected the response.** On the

* '(So) would you like to have a private doctor, if you could afford it, or would you rather keep an NHS one?'.

** 1964 'Are there some occasions when you would prefer to see a woman GP rather than a man?'. 1977 'Are there some occasions when you would prefer to see a doctor of a particular sex?'.

earlier study we did not ask men about their preference – a reflection of our changing attitudes!

The general picture is one of small variations between men and women and although the differences fell into the same patterns as in 1964 they were, if anything, less clear. Men seemed less attached to their own general practitioner, and with their somewhat greater orientation to the hospital, they may have felt less dependent on the general practitioner than did women. However women were not more likely to think they might discuss a personal problem with their doctor, nor that they would consult about a feeling of depression.

Age

As people become older they are more likely to be ill. Data from the General Household Survey 1977 show a marked rise in the proportion reporting chronic illness with increasing age. We only asked one question about health and this related to attitudes as people were asked whether they regarded their health *for their age* as excellent, good, fair, or poor. Replies are shown in *Table 89*. As might be expected when people were asked to take account of their age there were no definite trends but even so a higher proportion of older people, age 55 or more, rated their health as fair or poor for their age: 36% of them did so compared with 20% of those under 55.

Although, as we showed earlier in this chapter, association between age and consultation rates were not as marked as might have been expected there were two ways in which older people made a rather different use of the general practitioner service. People aged 55 or more were more likely to be taking some prescribed medicine during the two weeks before they were interviewed – 56% of them had done so compared with 30% of younger patients (Anderson, forthcoming). In addition as we showed earlier, in Chapter 3, home visiting increased with age, and 27% of people aged 75 or over compared with only 1% of people under that age said they never went to the surgery – the doctor always called.

Another factor besides ill-health which may lead to older people being more dependent on their doctor is that more of them live alone. The proportion of people in our sample who did so rose from 6% of those aged 18–54 to 15% of those aged 55–64 and to 33% of those aged 65 and over. Older people therefore have fewer potential

Table 89 Health rating by age

	Age								*All*
	18–20	*21–24*	*25–34*	*35–44*	*45–54*	*55–64*	*65–74*	*75+*	
Health for age, rated as:	%	%	%	%	%	%	%	%	%
Excellent	28	22	35	42	30	18	28	22	30
Good	53	49	49	37	47	41	40	45	44
Fair	19	26	15	17	20	28	24	27	21
Poor	—	3	1	4	3	13	8	6	5
Number of people (=100%)	32	59	171	139	131	135	102	63	835

supporters at home though they may be burdened with more ill-health. One indication that older people may see the doctor's role somewhat differently was that rather more of them thought a general practitioner was a suitable person to talk to about family problems: 35% of people aged 55 or more thought this against 27% of younger people, while the proportion who said that if they were worried about a personal problem that was not strictly medical they might discuss it with their general practitioner was 34% of those aged 55 or over, 25% of those under 55.

In a number of ways older people seem to have a rather closer relationship with their general practitioner than younger people but the position is complicated by the fact that, as we showed in Chapter 2, older people had been with their present doctor for longer and continuity of care was related to a number of aspects of the doctor-patient relationship. In terms of regarding their doctor as something of a personal friend both age and continuity of care seem important and they interact. It is older patients who have been with their doctor for some time who are most likely to describe their relationship with their doctor in this way. The proportion describing their doctor as a personal friend was 50% among patients aged 55 or more who had been with their doctor ten or more years, 27% for all others. Older people more often regarded their doctor as easy to talk to irrespective of the length of time they had been with him: the proportion describing their doctor as 'easy to talk to and ask questions' rose from 72% of those under 25 to 94% of those aged 65 or more. One difference that we had not expected was that older people were *less* likely to say they ever worried about wasting the doctor's time: there was a fall from 55% of those aged under 25 to 23% of those aged 65 or over in the proportion who worried about this. Given the differentials in reported ill-health between young and old and the much greater differentials in mortality, the differences in consultation rates seem smaller than might be expected on both our study and the General Household Survey. Even considering consultations by younger people for sickness certification and family planning it seems probable that older people are less likely to consult their doctor about minor problems. This is probably why they were less likely to worry about wasting the doctor's time.

There was quite a lot of evidence from our study that younger people had a less good relationship with their doctor. The proportion of people who described themselves as 'very satisfied' with the care they had received from their doctor increased from 42% of those aged 18–24 to 61% of those aged 65 and over. And younger people were more critical than older people about a number of aspects of their care. The proportions who said their doctor was 'not so good' about various aspects of their care are presented in *Table 90.*

Table 90 Age and the proportion of people who were critical of various aspects of their general practitioner care

	Age	
	18–54	*55+*
Proportion who felt their doctor was 'not so good' about:		
Having a pleasant, comfortable waiting room	36%	16%
Always visiting when asked	12%	6%
Sending people to hospital as soon as necessary	8%	3%
Keeping people waiting in waiting room	25%	10%
Examining people carefully and thoroughly	15%	6%
Taking time and not hurrying you	19%	7%
Listening to what you say	9%	2%
Explaining things to you fully	26%	14%
Number of people (=100%)	456	258

One reason for the generally higher level of criticism may be that younger people have higher expectations, particularly about information and communications. When asked: 'When you are ill do you like to know as much as possible about what is wrong with you or would you rather not know very much?' the proportion who said they wanted to know as much as possible fell from 91% of those under 45 to 75% of those aged 65 or more. In addition a higher proportion of younger people thought they were more likely to question the doctor than they were ten years ago – this proportion fell from 49% of those aged 25–34, to only 9% of people aged 65 or more. At the same time younger people were more likely to feel that the doctor's willingness to explain things had improved: 35% of those aged 25–54 thought their doctor was more likely to explain things adequately than he or she was ten years ago, but only 19% of older people felt this. Younger people were also more critical about communications between general practitioners and hospitals. The proportion who thought general practitioners knew too little about the treatment their patients got at hospital fell from 42% of people aged 18–24 to 21% of those aged 65 or more. Similarly, 53% of people aged 18–24 said that, when the general practitioner sent a patient to hospital the doctor at the hospital usually knew too little about the patient – only 25% of people aged 65 and over thought this.

Another possible reason for younger people being more critical is that they were not treated as well, particularly by receptionists. When asked how long they had waited the last time they went to the doctor's surgery 29% of people under 55 estimated that they had waited thirty minutes or longer, compared with 19% of older people. It may be that younger people are more likely to attend at peak times. Those under 55 were more likely to think a wait of half an hour or more unreasonable: 50% of them felt this, 27% of the older people who had been kept waiting that long – further evidence that expectations vary with age. There was no difference with age in the proportion whose doctor had an appointment system nor in the proportion who preferred an appointment system to waiting in turn.

On a number of issues it was the people under 35 who seemed to have the poorest relationship with the receptionists. Only 30% of them thought the receptionists were very helpful compared with 57% of older people and the proportions who thought the receptionists were helping them to get to the doctor were 56% of those under 35, 79% of those aged 35 or more. People under 35 did not report any greater delay than older people in getting an appointment, nor was there any difference by age in the proportions who were asked by the receptionist why they wanted to see the doctor. However 21% of those aged under 35 said that on at least one occasion in the last twelve months they had put off going to see the doctor because of the need for an appointment compared with only 8% of older people.

We have already suggested that older people may not consult their general practitioner as often as might be expected given their greater morbidity and mortality. It also appears that they were no more likely than younger people to go to hospital out-patient and casualty departments. The only difference that emerged was that 43% of people aged 18–35 had been to out-patients or casualty in the previous twelve months compared with 33% of older people.

(There were no significant differences between men and women over this.) Among those who had been, younger people were more likely to have gone directly, without being referred by their general practitioner: 37% of people under 35 attending out-patients or casualty had gone there directly compared with 21% of older attenders. Altogether younger people appeared more hospital-oriented – they more often predicted they would go direct to hospital in the event of either a cut leg needing stitching, or a fall at home during the day when they thought they might have a broken arm. The proportion who predicted they would go to hosptial with a cut leg declined from 87% of people aged 18–24, to 64% of those aged 65 and over; and the proportion who would call their general practitioner if they suspected a broken arm increased from 16% of people aged 18–24, to 35% of people aged 65 and over.

However there were no marked differences with age in the proportion who would prefer a system in which patients went straight to specialists or in the proportions who preferred a general practitioner who sent them to hospital for any tests. Nor were there any differences with age in the proportions who would like to have a private doctor if they could afford it or in the proportions preferring partnership to single-handed practice. So although younger patients were rather more critical and had somewhat different expectations they did not seem more likely to be looking for radical structural changes.

Social class

There were two reasons why middle-class patients might be expected to have rather less close relationships with their general practitioners than working-class patients. The first is that as a group, middle-class patients were slightly younger and we have just shown that older patients seemed more relaxed with their doctors and found them more approachable. Second, middle-class patients are much more mobile: there was a trend from 38% of people in Social Class I to 86% of those in Social Class V in the proportion who had lived in the same area for ten years or more, and the proportion who had been with the same doctor for ten years or more rose from 38% of Social Class I patients to 51% of those in Social Class V. Associated with these differences in age and mobility 24% of middle-class patients described their relationship with their doctor as friendly rather than businesslike compared with 37% of working-class people; and the proportions saying they knew their doctor 'very well' were 14% and 22% respectively.

In many ways the attitudes and reactions of middle- and working-class patients were similar. When asked what, if anything, they appreciated about their doctor similar proportions of middle- and working-class people mentioned personality qualities and there was no difference in the proportion describing attributes of their medical skills. About three-tenths of both groups mentioned a quality they thought a general practitioner ought to have that theirs had not got. There were no differences between middle- and working-class patients in the proportion who thought a general practitioner was a suitable person to talk to about family problems, nor were there any social class variations in people's assessments of their doctor about being good about examining them, keeping them waiting in the surgery, listening to what they said, and taking time and not hurrying them. Anxieties about wasting the doctor's time were also unrelated to class and there were no class differences in the proportion who said they had put off consulting the doctor because they felt the doctor was too busy or because of the need to make an appointment.

There were however a number of class differences in the way people used, or predicted they would use, the general practitioner service. Working-class patients were more likely than middle-class ones to say that if they were worried about a personal problem that was not strictly medical they would discuss it with their doctor: the proportions who would do so rose from 17% of those in Social Class I to 42% of those in Social Class V. In addition working-class patients were more likely to predict that they woud consult their doctor if they were depressed. Seventy-five per cent of them said they would do so compared with 63% of middle-class ones. We showed earlier that the proportion who had consulted their doctor (or his or her partners or locum) at all in the previous twelve months did not vary with social class, nor were there any class differences in the frequency of consultation for women, but working-class men saw their doctor rather more often than middle-class men. Over home visits there was a clear trend with the proportion of people who had received a home visit in the previous twelve months rising from 6% of those in Social Class I to 29% of those in Social Class V. This trend seems to be explained by differences in the proportion using private transport to get to the doctor's surgery. Both middle- and working-class patients were less likely to have a visit if they could go to the surgery by car and the differences between the middle- and working-class disappeared if the comparison was made between those using the same method of transport. Nevertheless as working-class patients are less likely to go to their doctors by private transport (the proportion who did so declined from 60% of people in Social Class I to 9% of those in Social Class V) they had more home visits and the proportion who said their doctor had never been to their home was 26% of middle-class patients, 20% of working-class ones. These differences were reflected in comments about this aspect of their care. One of the qualities in their doctors that they appreciated which was mentioned more frequently by working-class patients was the doctor's willingness to visit or that he or she visited promptly and without grumbling: 13% of the working-class patients made some favourable comment about this against 7% of middle-class patients. And when asked specifically whether they felt their doctor was 'good' about visiting when asked 75% of working-class people said this, 61% of middle-class. (More middle-class patients said they did not know, 29% compared with 15% of working-class patients, presumably because middle-class patients had less experience; there was no difference in the proportion describing their doctor as 'not so good' about this).

In contrast to home visits as a whole, it was the middle-class patients who were more likely to contact their doctor in an emergency. The proportion reporting that in the last twelve months they or their spouse had tried to get hold of the doctor in a hurry, in the evening, or at night for either themselves or their children fell from 23% of those in Social Class I to 6% of those in Social Class V. Possibly working-class patients are less confident that their doctor would be prepared to come out in an emergency; if so this could explain why a higher proportion of working-class patients preferred a deputizing service for night calls: 20% did so compared with 15% of middle-class patients.

So far the findings are similar to those on other studies (Earthrowl and Stacey 1977; Cartwright 1979) with few class differences in attitudes, and greater variations in the use of services. Over one aspect of care there were some differences in attitudes. Middle-class people seemed to want rather different sorts of information and explanation. When asked whether, when they were ill, they liked to know as much as possible about what was wrong with them, or whether they would rather not know very much, there were no differences between middle- and working-class patients; the great majority of all patients, 85%, said they wanted to know as much as possible, 10% said they would rather not know very much, the rest made other comments. But in response to a further question about whether they were basically interested in how the illness was going to affect them or whether they liked to know the actual mechanical details as well, 51% of the middle-class people said the latter compared with 42% of working-class people. With this difference it is perhaps surprising that middle-class people were no more (or less) likely to be critical of their doctor for not explaining things to them fully, or for not giving them an adequate explanation at their last consultation. However, working-class people appeared more appreciative of their doctor for explaining things in that 10% of them made some favourable comment about this when describing their doctor's qualities compared with only 5% of middle-class people. In addition, working-class people were more likely to think their doctor had improved in this respect: 32% of them said their doctors explained more now than they, or their predecessors, did ten years ago, but only 25% of middle-class patients thought this. Doctors almost certainly respond rather differently to middle- and working-class people. Other studies (Buchan and Richardson 1973; Cartwright and O'Brien 1976) have found that general practitioners spend rather longer talking to their middle-class than to their working-class patients. The higher expectations of middle-class patients may be met by longer consultations.

Middle-class patients may also have rather better doctors. There was some indication in the last chapter that people living in Conservative areas had doctors who could be thought of as 'better': they were more likely to have hospital appointments, to regard fewer of their consultations as trivial, to enjoy their work more, to consider consultations about family problems to be appropriate; and they were less likely to use a deputizing service. Similarly, middle-class people were more likely than those classified as working-class to have doctors with some of these characteristics; the differences are shown in *Table 91*.

The data suggest that middle-class patients were at an advantage in that they were more likely to have doctors with 'desirable'

Table 91 Social class of patients and some characteristics of their doctors

	Social class	
	Middle-class	*Working-class*
Proportion of their doctors:		
With a hospital appointment	46%	34%
Using deputizing service at all	35%	46%
Think it is appropriate to be consulted about family problems	72%	62%
With more than 3,000 patients (doctor's estimate)	34%	44%
With a further qualification	37%	29%
Qualified in a British medical school (excl. N. Ireland)	85%	77%
Whose practice has an ECG machine	46%	35%
Number of doctors (=100%)	222	276

attributes. Their doctors were more likely to have hospital appointments; to think it was appropriate to be consulted about family problems; to have a further qualification; to have qualified in a British medical school; to look after less than 3,000 patients; and to have an ECG machine. In addition doctors of middle-class people were less likely to use a deputizing service. However there were no significant differences between the doctors of working- and middle-class people in their access to beds, average number of procedures carried out, having an appointment system, training, age, membership of the Royal College of General Practitioners, enjoyment of general practice, or in the proportion of their consultations they thought were trivial.

One of the last questions we asked patients about their general practitioners was how satisfied on balance they felt with the care they had received from him or her. There was a clear trend from 35% of people in Social Class I to 64% of those in Social Class V in the proportion who described themselves as very satisfied. So our evidence suggests that working-class people, partly because of the length of time they have been with their doctors and partly because they have rather more home visits, have a somewhat closer relationship with their general practitioner in that they are more likely to consult him or her about psychological and social problems and they feel generally more satisfied with their care.

Turning to the use of hospital services we found no social class differences in the proportion who had been to hospital as an out-patient in the previous twelve months, nor in the proportion who had gone directly to casualty. The one class difference that did emerge was that a relatively low proportion of people in Social Classes IV and V had been to hospital as in-patients in the previous twelve months; 5% compared with 11% of those in other social classes. Another study (Cartwright 1979) showed that women in Social Class V were less frequently admitted to hospital during pregnancy. The findings from the two studies give a clear indication that the least privileged in relation to jobs and status are receiving less than their expected share of in-patient care.

There were no differences between middle- and working-class people in the proportion who said they would go straight to hospital with either a broken arm, or with a leg that needed stitching. Nor, in spite of their greater satisfaction with the care they had received from their general practitioner, were working-class patients any less (or more) likely to say they would rather go directly to a specialist than have a general practitioner as at present. If anything working-class people seemed to have more of a preference for hospital when tests and investigations were needed. Rather more of them, 46% compared with 32% of middle-class people, expressed a preference for the kind of general practitioner who sends patients to hospital if they need any investigation rather than one who did a number of tests and investigations at their surgery. And 8% of working-class people said their doctor was 'not so good' about 'sending people to hospital as soon as it was necessary' compared with 4% of middle-class people.

Finally, looking at class differences in attitudes to the National Health Service, we found that the proportion who approved of the idea was 75% of middle-class people, 81% of the working-class. Few, 2% of all patients, said they disapproved, the rest had mixed feelings. There were clear social class differences in the reasons for thinking the National Health Service was a good idea. Working-class people were more likely to emphasize personal advantages: the proportion saying they thought the National Health Service was a good idea because it allowed access to care without worries about costs, or who thought they could not otherwise afford care rose from

2% of professionals to 18% of unskilled people. Middle-class people, on the other hand, more often made comments with a societal emphasis: the proportion saying the National Health Service benefited those who could otherwise not afford to obtain care, or who said it was a fair system, giving equality of opportunity to receive necessary care fell from 36% of people in Social Class I to 18% of those in Social Class V. In spite of the rather lower level of approval for the National Health Service among the middle-class they were no more or less likely to say they would prefer to have a private doctor if they could afford one (29% of both groups said this). The proportion who had made some use of private medical care in the previous twelve months was 5% of the middle-class, 2% of the working-class (a difference which does not quite reach the 5% level of significance) while the proportions with some insurance for private medical care were 13% and 5% respectively.

To sum up, working-class people seem rather more appreciative of the care they get from their general practitioner although, when asked about specific aspects of care, there were hardly any social class differences in the level of criticism. Working-class patients may have a greater sense of loyalty to their doctor because they have been with the same doctor for longer, because the doctor is more likely to have visited their home, and because they may feel somewhat more dependent on him or her as they have fewer professional people to turn to in a family crisis. Middle-class patients, although they may have rather higher expectations in some ways, are no more critical about specific aspects of their care, possibly because they have rather better doctors, or doctors who treat them rather differently. The great majority of both middle- and working-class people support the idea of a National Health Service.

9 In conclusion

So, how do the experiences and views of patients and doctors in 1977 compare with those of their predecessors in 1964? This was the initial question we set out to explore.

In 1964 nearly everybody in this country had a general practitioner under the National Health Service. Most people had one they had known for several years, who was accessible, had been to their home at some time, and cared for other members of their family. The majority of patients were appreciative of this care. These considerable achievements had been generally maintained in 1977. What of the changes?

Few and small changes

The answer is in many ways disappointing since a number of improvements might have been not only hoped for but expected. In fact experiences and views had changed remarkably little. This is in spite of what might be seen as a considerable increase in investment of both money and manpower in general practice. Between the two studies payments to doctors for practice in groups, for vocational training, for out-of-hours responsibilities, for night visits, for employment of ancillary help, for rent and rates of premises, and for employment of locums during the doctor's own sickness had been introduced or substantially increased. These changes had led to the employment of many more secretaries and nurses in general practice, more group practices, and greatly increased attendances at post-graduate centres and courses. It might have been expected that this would lead to more contented doctors, a widening scope of activities in general practice, and a better relationship between patients and doctors. Our studies suggest that these expectations have not been realized. Possible reasons for this are discussed under three headings.

Doctor satisfaction

General practitioners in the two studies gave similar responses to a question about the extent to which they enjoyed their work. It is possible that this is because the question was too superficial or that responses reflect personality traits rather than the circumstances of their work. Job satisfaction is notoriously difficult to measure. Their descriptions of what they enjoyed about their work and what they found frustrating about it are possibly more illuminating. In 1977 more doctors said they enjoyed the diversity of their work and more expressed appreciation of their freedom and independence. There was a marked drop in the proportion complaining about inadequate leisure and being tied to their job but at the same time an increase in the proportion who said they felt frustrated because they did not have enough time to do their work properly. It may be that they are spending less time on the job and this has contributed to feelings about the pressure of work. In addition the majority of doctors felt they were more busy in 1977 than they had been ten years previously, or when they first went into practice, although we found little change in surgery consultation rates and a marked drop in home visits. The increase in secretaries, nurses, and other attached staff working with general practitioners may have enabled them to delegate some tasks, but coordinating the efforts of a team takes time and energy.

Other changes in society have inevitably influenced doctors' expectations about their leisure and working conditions. So if doctors were as satisfied or dissatisfied with their working conditions in 1977 as in 1964 this is almost certainly because conditions have improved and kept pace with rising expectations.

Prestige is one component of job satisfaction. Both doctors and patients thought that general practitioners' prestige in the community had fallen rather than risen but when asked about their prestige within the medical profession general practitioners thought it had gone up rather than down. Feelings about their prestige within the profession may be taken as an indication of professional morale and in 1964, before the Doctor's Charter, morale was at a low level. In 1977 we thought that the Charter, the influence of the Royal College of General Practitioners, and the emphasis on training would have given general practitioners a clearer sense of professional identity and more confidence, which in turn would lead to more satisfaction. In practice members of the Royal College of General Practitioners seemed to have a greater sense of professional identification than non-members. And it is possible that non-members found the increasing influence of the College, with its emphasis on whole-person medicine rather than traditional clinical practice, somewhat alienating. The same might apply to training schemes: a stimulus to those involved, a threat to those who were not. However neither College membership, training, nor attendance at courses related to statements about their enjoyment of their work. Again there may be effects which cancel out: some doctors gain stimulus and increased enjoyment in their work from further education and College membership, others go on courses or to College meetings to escape from a job which they are not enjoying.

Changes in the scope of general practice activities

There is no doubt that between 1964 and 1977 general practitioners became much more involved in giving advice and help about contraception. As a result more of them did vaginal examinations in the surgery. In addition general practitioners had better equipped surgeries and direct access to more hospital facilities in 1977 than in 1964. But that said, there is relatively little indication that the scope of their work has widened in other directions, and some indication that some procedures such as stitching cuts were less often done in the general practitioner's surgery at the later date. In spite of the large increase in the number of nurses working at general practitioner surgeries, and the fact that over a third of the doctors who worked with a nurse said that the nurse frequently did things that the patients would otherwise have to go to hospital for, there had been a substantial increase in the proportion of patients (from a quarter to a third) who said they had attended hospital out-patients or casualty departments in a year.

There are a number of ways in which the general practitioners' work might be seen as being more trivial in 1977 than in 1964.

During this time the proportion of babies born at home fell and the proportion of deaths occurring at home also declined. During the same period the number of hospital admissions rose while the average length of stay shortened. So the general practitioner became less involved in the major events of birth and death and possibly also with the acute phases of illnesses that were increasingly treated in hospital. In addition the general practitioner was doing less home visiting so may have cut himself or herself off from patients with chronic disabling illness. Furthermore because of the increasing use of deputizing services general practitioners were missing more of the emergencies in their practice.

One activity in which a decline might have been welcomed is prescribing. But in 1977 as in 1964 two-thirds of patients came away from the general practitioner's surgery with a prescription. Comparisons with another study in 1969 (Dunnell and Cartwright 1972) show that in both 1969 and 1977 over a third of adults had taken some prescribed medicine in the two weeks before the interview. By 1977 the cost of drugs was more than one-and-a-half times the cost of general medical services. Prescribing is not only a common activity of general practitioners, it is also an expensive one. As a society we pay less for the advice, the listening, the explaining, and the support that general practitioners give their patients than for the pharmaceutical products which they prescribe.

The doctor-patient relationship

One index of this from the doctors' viewpoint is the proportion of surgery consultations which they felt were trivial, inappropriate, or unnecessary. For doctors to regard a high proportion in this light suggests a degree of alienation from patients and their problems; a low proportion, a degree of identification. In 1964 the fact that a quarter of general practitioners considered at least half of their consultations to be trivial, inappropriate, or unnecessary was viewed with concern. It was found that to some extent doctors' feelings about 'triviality' seemed to be of their own making. Doctors who regarded a high proportion of consultations as trivial carried out few procedures themselves, had access to few diagnostic procedures, attended few courses, and were comparatively unlikely to express an interest in psychiatry. At the time it was thought that:

> 'An initial training, or a post-graduate training more orientated towards general practice should help future doctors; attendance at appropriate courses may help those at present in practice, but there is a danger that a spiral of cynicism, job-depreciation and anti-patient feeling has built up among some general practitioners and will be difficult to break down' (Cartwright 1967:62).

Thirteen years later, after the introduction of the general-practitioner training scheme and the enormous expansion of post-graduate education, it might have been hoped that there would have been a reduction in the proportion of consultations that general practitioners felt to be trivial, inappropriate, or unnecessary. But as we have seen there was no change. In 1977 as in 1964 there were a number of indications that doctors' attitudes and practices were associated with their perceptions about trivialities. In the later study doctors estimating a high proportion of consultations as trivial carried out fewer procedures themselves, were more likely to use a deputizing service, and were less likely to be trainers or members of the Royal College of General Practitioners, than their colleagues who regarded a smaller proportion of consultations as trivial. In addition patients were rather more critical of doctors who thought a lot of their consultations were trivial, for not taking time, and for hurrying them.

For a number of reasons that we have discussed earlier it could be argued that general practitioners might be more frustrated by trivialities in 1977 than in 1964. The observation that this does not appear to be so may be attributed to an improvement in other aspects of doctor-patient relationships, arising possibly from doctors' perceptions that patients in the last ten years have become more knowledgeable about health matters. However there are two ways in which doctor-patient relationships could be seen as deteriorating rather than improving or remaining static between 1964 and 1977. These are discussed next.

Deteriorations between 1964 and 1977

Both doctors and patients were less likely in 1977 than in 1964 to regard it as appropriate for patients to consult their general practitioner about problems in their family lives. At the same time many doctors felt there was a growing tendency for people to look to them for this sort of help. Acknowledgement of this broader role was shown to be associated with doctors' enjoyment of their work and to their estimates of the proportion of trivial consultations. So a decrease in the proportion of doctors who accept that giving support to patients with family problems is part of their job is likely to lead to an increase in discontent among doctors as well as a cut back in the range of help that is given to patients. We are not saying that we want general practitioners to take on the role of social workers or that patients should see the general practitioner as the appropriate person to consult about all their family problems. But we would hope that general practitioners, sensitive to the social content of many medical problems and recognizing the special status as trusted adviser they have for many patients, would be willing to help patients, possibly by referral, when approached about such problems. Again it might have been hoped that more specific training for general practice might have encouraged them to widen rather than to restrict their interest and activities in this field. The observation that general practitioners seem to be less willing to do so will be a disappointment to many trainers as well as to teachers in social medicine and academic departments of general practice.

The other aspect of the general practitioner service that has deteriorated from the patients' viewpoint is home visiting. This has declined and patients' criticisms over this increased four-fold between the two studies. Some fall in the extent of home visiting from the 1964 level was possibly reasonable and an inevitable result of the increase in the proportion of the population with access to a motor car. But the fall was greater than would have been expected from this fact alone and we have shown, and others such as Gray (1978) have argued persuasively from individual experience, that fewer home visits often mean a deterioration in doctor-patient relationships. Doctors know and understand less about the patients' backgrounds and circumstances, while patients probably reveal less of themselves, their fears, and their courage in the intimidating surroundings of the surgery than in the familiarity of their homes. Moreover the fall in the proportion of patients who are visited relatively frequently suggests that doctors are visiting the chronically ill or disabled less often. Doctors may argue that community nurses in 1977 were doing some of the tasks that the doctors would have had to do in 1964 but our study shows that patients are not happy with the cut back in personal contact with the doctor. Nurses may be able to carry out various procedures and give help and care at one level but it may be that the chronically ill and disabled feel the need for some regular contact with and support from their doctor.

The deterioration in the service indicated by doctors' unwillingness to accept the social content of their work and the lack of improvement in attitudes to 'trivial' consultation are more surprising because it would seem from reading the Journal of the Royal College of General Practitioners and the writings of doctors in academic departments of general practice that more emphasis and attention is being placed on learning to care, and less on a mechanistic model. (See for example McCormick 1979). But doctors who are vocal in the press and at universities are likely to be atypical and a picture of their attitudes will give a mistaken impression of a renaissance in general practice. Our 1977 study covered a representative sample in terms of basic characteristics such as age, sex, and type of practice but it is confined to the two-thirds who were prepared to answer our questions so it may have other biases. However it is probable that the research-minded as well as trainers and College members were more likely to respond to our survey and these will be the ones most exposed to the views of the proselytizers and academic leaders. So the views of those at the grass roots having little contact or experience of recent post-graduate education and those rejecting the views of their trainers and leaders may well be under-represented.

Our study indicates that in at least two ways general practitioners are retreating from more intimate contacts with their patients. The total picture may well be more gloomy than our study suggests.

Improvements between 1964 and 1977

The main improvement, in our view, has been that in 1977 patients were more willing to criticize their doctor and to question what the doctor did or said. It seemed that patients were more knowledgeable about health matters in 1977 than they were in 1964 and this seems to have led to more self-confidence and less passive acceptance. In many spheres of life authority is questioned more openly, paternalism accepted less readily. But amongst patients, like doctors, the most vocal may not be widely representative.

It is easy to exaggerate the size of the change. Our surveys show that it is there, but it is small. And the effect of such changes in patients' attitudes is likely to be even smaller, particularly in times of economic cut-backs on the health services. Very few, less than 2% of patients in 1977, were aware that there was an organization, the Community Health Council, that aimed to represent the views of local users of the health services to the health authorities (Anderson 1979), and this limited channel of influence is currently under threat (DHSS and Welsh Office 1979).

We welcome the evidence that patients are less passive, partly because we view an uncritical acceptance as being conducive to stagnation and apathy, and partly because we see the changes as leading to an improvement in patient-doctor relationships. We think these relationships are gradually becoming more equal with patients able to communicate their needs and desire for information more directly and doctors willing to respond more openly. If doctors are more willing to reveal the limits of their knowledge and capabilities this is likely to make patients' expectations more realistic and lead to a greater understanding and mutual respect.

One indication of the sort of change that may be developing is that patients are becoming more suspicious of and reluctant to take drugs. Again the change is small but it is there. It may be difficult for patients to convey this to doctors without appearing to reject an offer of help. Most patients are sensitive to doctors' feelings and reluctant to upset their doctor. But it is much easier to communicate a positive than a negative desire. So doctors may be unaware when patients do not want drugs, but will generally realize it when they do. They get a mistaken impression about the proportion of patients who desire drugs. This leads to one of our three immediate practical suggestions.

Three suggestions

Some general practitioners, in situations where a drug might be of marginal help, have adopted a policy of asking patients whether they want a prescription or not. They report that they have been surprised at the numbers who have said they do not want one. We would like to see more doctors adopting this policy, and would predict that it might in time lead to a substantial decrease in prescribing. Thomas (1978) has shown that patients tolerate no treatment better than doctors think they will. While Marsh (1977) presents evidence that with a system involving more explanation a considerable reduction in prescribing can be made. He found patients to be well aware of iatrogenic diseases and pleased to see attempts made to prevent it.

Our second straightforward suggestion relates to receptionists and stems from our finding that a substantial proportion of patients did not feel it was appropriate for receptionists to ask them why they wanted to see the doctor. The practice appeared to lead to ill-feeling between patients and receptionists and to create a barrier between patients and doctors. So our suggestion is that receptionists should *not* ask patients seeking an appointment what is wrong with them. They should ask patients when they would like to come, tell them when the next routine appointment is available, and explain that there is an arrangement for fitting in emergencies. Some doctors will want to keep a time at the end of their appointments when people who want to see him or her urgently can be seen without a previous appointment. Others will want to keep some appointment spaces unfilled until the last minute in case emergencies turn up. Whatever the system, doctors and receptionists need to discuss it from time to time and tell each other how well it is working from their point of view. It is important that receptionists should feel comfortable about the arrangement, otherwise their discontents are likely to be communicated to the patients.

Third, and as in 1964 we would like to see a change in the arrangements for sickness certification. The present system leads to frustration for doctors and patients and can create tension between them. As McCormick (1979:79–81) says the doctor's role in this is an unhappy one: 'Society demands that he distinguish the malingerer from the genuinely ill. In practice this is a totally unreal expectation and he has virtually no option but to endorse the individual's decision to be sick.' Gardner (1979) puts it more strongly: 'The time has come to admit quite openly that medical certificates are, for all practical purposes, issued on demand. Some doctors and many managers believe that control can be exerted by medical certification, but all available studies indicate the futility of this approach.' For patients too the situation is unsatisfactory. Faced, for example, with a feverish cold needing a couple of days in bed the patient can drag himself to the surgery to his discomfort and the detriment of the other patients, or irritate the doctor by asking for a home visit or by turning up at the surgery asking for a retrospective certificate for an illness which has passed. And the need to obtain a certificate for short-term sickness absence may engender the view that consultation is appropriate for minor illness. The BMA is seeking the abolition of social security certificates for periods of incapacity of three days or less. This in itself might remove some of the irritations and frustrations on both sides. It would seem to us that a more radical change is appropriate and that responsibility for reporting sickness absence to employers and National Insurance should normally belong to patients themselves. Sickness absence would not necessarily increase and might decline.

More fundamental comments

Our more fundamental comments are stimulated by our findings but do not derive just from them. They arise from our observations and readings, and they depend on our values and opinions. So we should make it explicit that we believe in a National Health Service and agree with the recent Royal Commission that it should:

> 'encourage and assist individuals to remain healthy; provide equality of entitlement to health services; provide a broad range of services of a high standard; provide equality of access to these services; provide a service free at the time of use; satisfy the reasonable expectations of its users; remain a national service responsive to local needs.'

We also agree with the Commission that 'compared with most other countries we have an extremely well-developed primary care system and we would be foolish to allow it to deteriorate.'

Our comments are therefore directed towards ways in which these aims of the NHS could be furthered. They relate to medical education, the definition of the general practitioner's role, the role of the Royal College of General Practitioners in this, team care, and the role of nurses and social workers in primary health care.

Medical education

The Royal Commission on Medical Education reported in 1968, four years after our first study. They described 'the increasing frustration and dissatisfaction of many general practitioners at their inability to deal with the substantial proportion of patients whose difficulties are psychological or social in origin and the alleged inability of many specialists to regard the patient as a person rather than as a case of a particular disease.' Most of the doctors in our

1977 study received their undergraduate medical training before the recommendations of the Commission on training in general practice and the behavioural sciences were made, let alone implemented, so we could not expect them to be influenced by the Todd proposals. But in any case we doubt if the report gave enough emphasis to training in the community. It recommended that 'every undergraduate medical student should be given an insight into general practice' and described how 'in some medical schools undergraduate students are attached for a few weeks to selected general practitioners, sitting in their surgeries and accompanying them on visits' but it did not lay down in detail any particular scheme. Around two-fifths of medical students are likely to spend most of their working lives in general practice; alongside this a few weeks out of a five-year undergraduate course appears paltry.

It seems to us that more radical changes are needed. Marinker (1974) has described the way students assimilate the ethos of medicine during the training in teaching hospitals and he recognized the 'hidden curriculum' of medical education – the values that teachers impart to their students. We do not feel the proposals of the Commission go far enough to counteract the influence of the hospital. For undergraduates one way to redress the balance might be a general shift towards the policy adopted in those medical schools which put considerable emphasis on practice in the community and expose their students to a variety of situations outside the hospital throughout their medical education. This could benefit those whose subsequent careers are in the hospital as well as those who opt for work outside. It should increase awareness of conditions in the community and of the other services there and facilitate understanding between the different services. But this still takes the basic training for hospital doctors as the starting point and we would like to see even more fundamental changes considered – medical schools whose basic aim is to train general practitioners.

The proliferation of *vocational training schemes* for trainee general practitioners has been one of the main developments in medical education in the last ten years. Freeman and Byrne (1973) have made a number of assessments from which they conclude that there is good evidence for the implementation of vocational training. However, as they point out, Peterson and others (1956) found that substantial differences between trained and untrained physicians tended to narrow and almost disappear over time. Freeman and

Byrne's assessments of training programmes showed improvements in 'clinical factual recall' and 'problem-solving skill in patient management.' They say that work is in hand to examine whether these improvements are maintained over any length of time. Their findings on any changes in attitude have yet to be published. Our study showed that trainers differed from other doctors in their opinions about a number of aspects of their work, but doctors who had spent a trainee year in general practice were no more likely than other doctors to share the trainer's views. Freeman and Byrne also found 'highly significant differences between trainers and trainees in . . . tests which examined the capacity to define a patient's problems, to undertake management and therapy, and to relate with patients and colleagues.' In our view the long-term value of these schemes is still to be demonstrated. Attitudes formed over a long period in medical school with its emphasis on hospital-oriented medical care are likely to be difficult to change and attendance at courses for *continuing education* may provide the occasion for them to be reinforced by discussion with other colleagues and hospital doctors with similar views.

There was a substantial increase from 1964 to 1977 in the proportion of general practitioners attending courses and it might have been hoped that this would have helped to prevent the development of cynicism and feelings of isolation among general practitioners that were noted in the 1964 study. But doctors' feelings that a high proportion of consultations are trivial, inappropriate, or unnecessary is probably a good indication of cynicism about their work and this had not altered. One of the basic difficulties over continuing education is to achieve a reasonable balance of courses for individual doctors so that their skills and knowledge are extended and their ideas can be challenged. A good range of courses can stimulate professionally and raise morale. But there is a danger that financial inducements can sometimes have a depressing effect, attracting the unenthusiastic and so creating an atmosphere of resistance to ideas which challenge accepted viewpoints and comfortable entrenched beliefs. A parallel danger is that of preaching to the converted, with courses that attract like-minded doctors with similar beliefs which are then reinforced rather than critically examined. Possibly financial inducements to attend courses should go hand in hand with some supervision and direction over the selection of courses attended.

So altogether we are somewhat sceptical about existing methods and schemes for undergraduate, post-graduate, and continuing education to break away from the domination of the hospital in medical education and in patterns of medical care. Some existing schemes may be attempting this but their efforts seem too little and too late.

Definition of the role of the general practitioner and the role of the Royal College of General Practitioners

Another conclusion from the 1964 study was that: 'The most obvious flaw in the organisation of the general practitioner service . . . is the uncertainty about the doctor's role.' Horder (1977) discussing the relationship between physicians and family doctors argued that specialists and general practitioners should have clearly defined and distinct functions. Clarification of the general practitioner's role has been a concern of the Royal College of General Practitioners who have accepted the following definition (Leeuwenhorst Working Party 1977):

> 'The general practitioner's specific role is to care for any human being as a whole person in his own environment; his concern goes beyond the requirements of a particular "incident" of illness. He interprets the patient's needs and demands in biological and pathological as well as in social and psychological terms. He provides continuity of care, irrespective of the numbers of incidents or types of illness that the patient may encounter.
>
> He differs from those in other fields of practice in that he does not restrict his work to any particular part or system of the human body, or to any particular form of prevention, diagnosis or treatment, or to a group of patients specified by age, sex or disease.
>
> The general practitioner is a licensed medical graduate who gives personal, primary and continuing care to individuals, families and a practice population, irrespective of age, sex and illness. It is the synthesis of these functions which is unique. He will attend his patients in his consulting room and in their homes and sometimes in a clinic or a hospital. His aim is to make early diagnoses. He will include and integrate physical, psychological and social factors in his considerations about health and illness. This will be

expressed in the care of his patients. He will make an initial decision about every problem which is presented to him as a doctor. He will undertake the continuing management of his patients with chronic, recurrent or terminal illnesses. Prolonged contact means that he can use repeated opportunities to gather information at a pace appropriate to each patient and build up a relationship of trust which he can use professionally. He will practice in co-operation with other colleagues, medical and non-medical. He will know how and when to intervene through treatment, prevention and education to promote the health of his patients and their families. He will recognise that he also has a professional responsibility to the community.'

These general formulations are useful as statements of principles but we think a more specific job description is needed which could be used to identify learning objectives for educational programmes and would also provide a basis for the imposition of minimum standards. The Birmingham Research Unit of the Royal College of General Practitioners (1977) has described a way of carrying out a continuous clinical and administrative self-audit or self-evaluation which could be used as the basis for a more specific job description. The Unit proposes that the findings of self-audits from group practices should be accumulated and available to other groups. The findings should be the basis for information about clinical performance. The audits could relate to equipment, use of ancillary help and of diagnostic tests, consultation times, as well as to prescribing patterns for different types of drugs and to the nature and frequency of different sorts of referral. The job or profile, would be constantly reassessed and amended with changes in circumstances and developments in health care.

The College itself favours self-assessment: 'The College understands the need to help individual doctors to identify their own educational and operational weaknesses through self-assessment, an approach much less threatening than a statutory review' (Council of the Royal College of General Practitioners 1974).

Medical schools with a particular interest in primary care could stimulate and assist groups to carry out such audits. These evaluations will also contribute to monitoring the quality of care in general practice. As Stevens (1977) maintains: it *can* be assessed, and better instruments to do this must be developed. 'To do these things will be difficult; not to do them would be unthinkable.'

There is still the problem of the application of the standards that have been defined being applied to professionally isolated general practitioners and professionally insulated partnerships who are not prepared to undergo even the limited rigours of self-assessment. Only about a quarter of general practitioners are members of the Royal College of General Practitioners so its influence is limited. But if the regulation of standards is to be left with the medical profession some body or bodies need the expertise to lay down appropriate standards and the motivation and the power to enforce them.

The threat of litigation is, as McCormick (1979) says, an unhappy method of seeking control but with patients becoming more knowledgeable and rather more critical they may well become more litigious if the profession itself does not do more to maintain acceptable standards of professional competence and to ensure that patients are not occasionally exposed to care from the indolent, the inept, or those who are physically or mentally unfit. To quote the Royal College of General Practitioners (1974) again: 'The profession wishes to be allowed to exercise discipline over its own members and to maintain its own standards in teaching and research. Thus, there must be a fair and just balance between professional freedom and a regulation that ensures high standards of care for patients.' How that regulation is to be achieved is a question that cannot be left to the professions indefinitely without a clear and satisfactory answer.

Team care and the role of nurses and social workers in primary health care

There have been many descriptions and analyses of different types of collaboration between nurses and general practitioners (see Marsh and Kaim-Caudle 1976). One difficulty is that, as Jefferys (1976) has pointed out: 'Innovations have a way of being successful because innovators are thoughtful people with charisma and enthusiasm.' It is another area in which careful evaluation is needed, but the evidence that nurses are accepted as playing a useful role in primary care is encouraging. Patients in general are conservative, apprehensive about change but adapting to it and then accepting it. Nurses working in the surgery have been a relatively welcome innovation to patients and doctors. Both recognize surgery nurses as an advantage. But are their skills and knowledge being used in the most appropriate way, or, to pose the question rather differently, are their knowledge and skills the most appropriate ones?

A study by Bowling (in press) revealed considerable uncertainty among both nurses and doctors about the nurses' role in the surgery, in the community, and in relation to the initial screening of patients. A division of labour between doctors and nurses in a way which makes the maximum use of their skills may conflict with the goal of continuity of care for patients. Some nurses prefer to work under supervision; others seek autonomy. And the extent to which doctors are willing and able to take on management responsibilities in a primary health care team also varies.

There are many ways in which these uncertainties might be resolved. Flexibility is needed. One approach we would like to see explored is for some fully trained nurses to be given more autonomy over *caring* than they have in most general practice situations. This seems to be the particular contribution that fully trained nurses have to make in primary care, as in hospital. And there is some evidence that general practice needs strengthening in this field, particularly in relation to the old and the disabled. We would like to see these nurses taking decisions about which patients need nursing care, and not relying on referrals from hospitals and general practitioners to determine this. Patients and their families would be able to approach these primary care nurses directly to ask for nursing care. The nurses would be working with, not for, doctors. They would be able to refer patients to doctors and they might be able to delegate some of the specific tasks to less skilled people. We would also like to see more experiments with nurses carrying out screening programmes, visiting old people in the practice who had not contacted the doctor or nurse or about whom little was known. Doctors would refer patients to them in the same way as they would refer patients to other doctors. Nurses and doctors would act as independent professional people and this could play a useful and important part in the monitoring of the care given both by nurses and doctors.

Another potential field for experiment is the extent and nature of the training needed by people undertaking technical tasks at the surgery under the supervision of doctors. Short courses for specific tasks might be most appropriate.

The role of social workers in primary health care teams seems to us more problematic, but the link between general practice and the social services is one of the most unsatisfactory aspects of our health and social services. Reorganization may have widened rather than narrowed the gap, and we need an overlap not a gap. Although our study suggests that attachment of social workers can do something to improve relations between the two services it also shows that even when such attachments exist the relationship is still often far from satisfactory. Something more radical is needed. Local schemes to facilitate liaison between all the different services concerned with the welfare of children, the elderly, the disabled, and the mentally ill need careful evaluation.

Financial arrangements

Our comments and suggestions up to now have concentrated on the things that seem to us to need changing. That seemed the most positive and constructive approach. But there is one possible change that we would *not* like to see – towards a wider use of fee for service. It can be argued that doctors' feelings about consultations for what they see as trivial, inappropriate, or unnecessary reasons relate simply to the way doctors are paid. If doctors were paid for each consultation they would not mind and might even welcome such undemanding and unworrying contacts. So an item of service payment would reduce doctors' frustrations on this score and by removing this source of irritation it might improve doctor-patient relationships. There may be some truth in this argument and there is some evidence that demands for a change to fee for service methods of payment are more likely to come from doctors who regard a high proportion of their consultations as trivial (Anderson, in draft). But the disadvantages of the fee for service arrangement in our view far outweigh such a possible advantage. In brief, it would seem that a fee for service system tends to encourage inappropriate and possibly harmful patterns of care and increase the cost of health services to the detriment of patients (Wolfe and Badgely 1974). The Royal Commission on the National Health also opposed the extension of item of service payments in general practice (except possibly for preventive measures) on the grounds that they distort patterns of service and may be expensive.

Finally, one major advantage of our system is that it is a dynamic one. It has changed in many ways in the last thirteen years. This ability to develop to meet changing needs and rising expectations is vital. We hope our study has signposted the way to further changes that will benefit both patients and their doctors.

Appendix I
The Study Areas

The study areas were parliamentary constituencies. To select our sample all constituencies were divided first into three groups: county constituencies, borough constituencies, and Welsh constituencies. Within each group constituencies were listed by county (pre-1974 arrangements) on a north to south basis and within county alphabetically. The number of parliamentary electors in each constituency was also listed and summed cumulatively. To choose the twenty constituencies for our study the grand total of electors in all constituencies was divided by twenty to give a sampling interval, x. A starting point, y, less than x, was taken from a book of random numbers. Then taking the cumulative totals of electors in the constituencies, those in which the numbers y, y + x, y + 2x, y + 3x, etc. fell were selected for the sample.

So we had a sample of areas selected after stratification by type of constituency and by region with probability proportional to the number of electors. They are shown in *Table A*.

Nine of the twenty returned a Labour member to parliament in October 1974 and eleven a Conservative. Density was much higher in the borough constituencies than in the county ones.

Another way in which areas can be classified is by whether they are 'designated' – that is, more doctors are encouraged to move into them because list sizes are large – intermediate or restricted, where there are certain restrictions on new doctors moving in because list sizes are low, and open areas where doctors are not restricted but there is no particular financial incentive. Doctors were classified by the DHSS as having practices in one of these four types of area and for the most part the majority of doctors in each of our study areas were classed as working in the same type of area. Labour constituencies were generally designated or open areas while Conservative constituencies were mostly restricted or intermediate ones.

Table A Study Areas

	County	*Voting October 1974 election*	*Density (electors per hectare)**	*Main type of area*
County constituencies:				
Workington	Cumberland	Labour	0.79	Intermediate/ Restricted
Hemsworth	Yorkshire	Labour	4.54	Open
W. Derbyshire	Derbyshire	Conservative	0.63	Intermediate/ Restricted
Stratford on Avon	Warwickshire	Conservative	0.76	Intermediate
Bedford	Bedfordshire	Conservative	2.54	Designated
Harlow	Essex	Labour	6.27	Open
Farnham	Surrey	Conservative	3.16	Intermediate
Royal Tunbridge Wells	Kent	Conservative	2.17	Intermediate
Shoreham	Sussex	Conservative	2.44	Intermediate
Borough constituencies:				
Burnley	Lancashire	Labour	27.81	Open
St. Helens	Lancashire	Labour	21.26	Designated
Pudsey	Yorkshire	Conservative	11.17	Intermediate
Nottingham North	Nottinghamshire	Labour	33.86	Designated
Birmingham Yardley	Warwickshire	Labour	34.55	Open

Enfield Southgate	London	Conservative	24.48	Restricted
Lambeth Streatham	London	Conservative	68.58	Intermediate
City of Westminster, Paddington	London	Labour	108.95	Restricted
Thanet East	Kent	Conservative	18.43	Open
Wales				
Monmouth	Monmouthshire	Conservative	0.78	Intermediate

* From Office of Population Censuses and Surveys, Electoral Statistics 1977.

Table B Types of area

	Labour	*Conservative*	*Total*
Designated or Open	7	2	9
Intermediate or Restricted	2	9	11
Total	9	11	20

Appendix II
The selection and response of patients

For our sample of patients or potential patients fifty people were taken from the electoral register in each of the twenty study areas. This was done on a systematic basis with a random starting point.

The combination of taking equal numbers from the chosen constituencies and choosing the constituencies with probability proportional to the number of electors means that we have a 'random' sample – in the sense that each person on an electoral register in England and Wales had an equal chance of being included.

Interviewers tried to contact all the 1,000 people selected in this way. We were anxious not to lose people who had moved, so if the person selected had moved but other members of his or her household were still living at the original address, the interviewer tried to find out where the person was now living and we contacted them there if it was possible. If the house or flat was empty the interviewer tried to find out where the person had moved from neighbours or other people in the area. If the person and all those living in the same household had moved and another household had moved into that house or flat, then the interviewer found out who was living there now and selected a person from that new household in a way that was laid down beforehand and led to an unbiased selection.*

In fact 31 people were 'substituted' in this way, but another 39 were no longer living at the address on the register and could not be traced or no substitute was interviewed. Twenty-eight people were followed up to another address and interviewed there. So we were only successful in replacing or following up three-fifths of those 10% of people who were not living at the address where they were listed. But the most common reason

* Precise details are in the *Notes for Interviewers*. These may be obtained from the Institute at 14 South Hill Park, London NW3. There will be a charge for photocopying.

for not obtaining an interview was a refusal. One out of ten of the initial sample and a quarter of those identified as substitutes were not prepared to answer our questions.

How important are these failures? The age, sex, and marital status of our sample are compared with figures for England and Wales (Central Statistical Office 1979) in *Table C*. The distributions are similar although our sample contains a relatively low proportion of people aged 18–24 – a mobile group who can be hard to trace and persuade to participate in surveys.

Table C Age, sex, and marital distributions of our sample compared with the population in England and Wales

	Study sample	*England and Wales*
Age:	%	%
18–24	10.9	13.6
25–34	20.7	19.4
35–44	16.7	15.5
45–54	15.7	16.1
55–64	16.2	15.5
65–74	12.2	12.6
75 or more	7.6	7.3
*Sex**:	%	%
Male	48.6	47.6
Female	51.4	52.4
*Marital Status**:	%	%
Sigle	15.1	15.1
Married	71.5	71.7
Widowed	11.1	10.3
Divorced	2.3	2.9
Number of people aged 18 or more (=100%)*	830	35,920

* Marital status and sex of people in England and Wales is based on those aged 20 and over.

Appendix III
The sample of doctors

All but seventeen of the people we interviewed gave us the name of their doctor. These 819 people told us about 543 doctors. For five of the patients it was a private doctor and for seventy-six it was a partner of the doctor whose National Health Service list they were on because they felt they knew the partner better and regarded him or her as their doctor. The number of people reporting the same doctor is shown in *Table D*.

Table D Number of patients reporting the same doctor

Survey patients with same doctor	*Number of doctors*	*Number of patients*
1	347	347
2	144	288
3	32	96
4	14	56
5	4	20
6	2	12
Total	543	819

Three hundred and sixty-five of the 543 doctors, 67%, completed a questionnaire. Most of the others just did not reply even after two reminders, but 4% wrote refusing to take part and 2% had died, retired, or were too ill.

A number of facts about both the doctors who replied and those who did not were obtained from the DHSS. These related to their age, type of practice, and country of qualifications. Information about members of the Royal College of General Practitioners was obtained from the College, and

Table E Variations in the proportion of doctors who responded

	Proportion of doctors who responded	*Number of doctors approached (=100%)*
Date of birth:		
Before 1916	63%	72
1917–1926	66%	180
1927–1936	71%	170
1937 or later	70%	104
Sex:		
Male	69%	474
Female	65%	57
Country of qualification:		
Great Britain	70%	425
Eire or N. Ireland	61%	44
Asia	53%	45
Elsewhere	(80%)	15
Qualification:		
Licentiate only	55%	77
University degree	68%	278
Some further qualification	73%	177
Trainer:		
Yes	84%	37
No	67%	491
Number of partners:		
Single-handed	61%	82
Two	64%	128
Three	69%	159
Four	78%	94
Five or more	70%	60
Member of Royal College of General Practitioners:		
Yes	78%	90
No	66%	442
Average list size of partnership:		
Less than 1,500	64%	28
1,500–1,999	77%	75
2,000–2,499	68%	164
2,500–2,999	68%	148
3,000 or more	64%	107
Type of area:		
Designated	63%	91
Open	67%	141
Intermediate	70%	203
Restricted	72%	90

information about qualifications from the Medical Register. The response rates of doctors in the various categories are shown in *Table E.*

There was some suggestion that as in 1964 and other Institute studies, (Dunnell and Cartwright 1972; Cartwright 1970) older doctors were less likely to reply than younger doctors and those in single-handed practice less likely than those in partnerships, but in this study the observed differences did not reach a level of statistical significance. Response rates for men and women doctors were similar. Doctors who qualified in Asia were comparatively unlikely to respond. The better qualified and the more professionally involved doctors, in the sense that they were appointed trainers or members of the Royal College of General Practitioners, had comparatively high response rates. The small trend in response rates with type of area did not reach a level of statistical significance.

Comparisons of patients' attitudes to doctors who responded and those who did not showed few differences. One that reached a level of significance was their assessment of their relationship as friendly or businesslike. Response rates were slightly higher when the patients rated the relationship as businesslike, 70%, than when they described it as friendly, 60%. A businesslike attitude may encompass the completion of questionnaires!

Apart from the bias arising because a third of the doctors did not participate in the study, there is the complication that the chance of a doctor being included in the sample is related to the number of patients who regard him or her as their doctor. *Table F* shows first the number of patients the doctors in our sample estimated they looked after,* and compares this with the proportion of patients in our sample who had doctors looking after these numbers of patients. In practice these two distributions were almost identical. Even so, doctors who looked after 3,000 patients had twice as much chance of being included in our study as doctors looking after 1,500

Table F Number of patients the doctors looked after

	Participating doctors	*Patients' doctors*	*Estimate of all doctors*
Number of patients:	%	%	%
Under 1,500	3	2	5
1,500–1,999	8	7	12
2,000–2,499	23	23	26
2,500–2,999	29	29	27
3,000 or more	37	39	30
Number of doctors (= 100%)	348	519	

* 'What is the approximate number of patients on your list? If in partnership, please estimate the number of NHS patients that you look after to the nearest 100.'

patients, so in order to estimate the proportion of all doctors looking after different numbers we have weighted the figures in the first column. This reduces the proportions looking after large numbers of patients slightly but the differences between the distributions are not large.

In the report analyses have been done on the sample of patients' doctors when characteristics of patients are related to those of doctors. For simplicity, and because the bias is small, the unweighted sample of participating doctors is used for analyses which involve doctors only.

It is possible to check the representativeness of both our initial sample and our sample of participating doctors by comparing them with information about all doctors in England (DHSS 1977a) for a few characteristics. *Table G* shows that the distributions by number of partners

Table G Comparison of our sample of doctors with national figures

	Sample selected	*Partici-pating doctors*	*All doctors in England 1976*
Type of partnership:	%	%	%
Single handed	16	14	17
Partnership of 2	24	23	20
3	31	30	24
4	18	21	19
5	4	5	11
6+	7	7	9
Type of area:	%	%	%
Designated	17	16	15
Open	27	26	30
Intermediate	39	40	39
Restricted	17	18	16
Age:	%	%	%
Under 30	3	3	7
30–39	17	18	24
40–49	32	33	28
50–59	34	33	26
60–69	12	11	12
70 or more	2	2	3
Sex:	%	%	%
Male	89	90	85
Female	11	10	15
Number of doctors (=100%)	523	356	*

* Data on partnerships and type of area are based on 20,551 unrestricted principles, those on age and sex on all 22,015 medical practitioners.

and by type of area were reasonably comparable although doctors in partnerships of three were somewhat over-represented in our initial and participating samples. But younger doctors, under 40, were apparently under-represented in our initial sample and among those who responded and so were women doctors. These differences may arise because assistants and trainees are included in the Department's figures for these characteristics.

We can also compare the proportion of doctors in our sample who were members of the Royal College of General Practitioners with data from the College about membership. College data indicate that membership in Great Britain is around 25% compared with only 17% in our initial sample. However, College figures include a number of doctors who have retired, they cover Scotland which has a relatively high proportion of members, and their membership is relatively low in conurbations (Norell, personal communication).

Finally information collected from the doctors in the survey can be compared with data relating to these same doctors from DHSS records. This gives some indication of the validity of our data. But most of the DHSS data relate to October 1976* whereas the doctors were approached in the summer of 1977 so there may be some discrepancies because of the time gap.

Where information was available from the two sources it tallied over whether or not the doctor was a trainer in 92% of cases but this apparently high level of agreement hides a considerable discrepancy since there were relatively few trainers: 9% according to the DHSS, 16% according to the doctors. Twenty-seven of the twenty-nine discrepancies were in the same direction – reported as trainers by the doctors but not by the Department. This may be because of the rapidly increasing number of recognized trainers.

Over health centres there was also a 92% agreement, and here too most of the discrepancies, twenty-eight out of thirty, were in the same direction with more doctors stating that they worked in health centres.

When the number of partners is considered there is more scope for discrepancies as six different categories were compared. The level of total agreement was 81% and within one doctor it was 96%. Discrepancies were more evenly divided, forty doctors reporting a larger number of partners than the Department recorded and twenty-seven fewer.

* Data about health centres and about group practice allowance relate to the summer of 1977.

Appendix IV
Statistical significance and sampling errors

There are a number of factors, particularly the nature of the data and the stage at which precise hypotheses were often formulated, that violate some of the conditions in which statistical tests of significance apply and make interpretation difficult. For this reason they are rarely referred to in the text, in an attempt to avoid the appearance of spurious precision which the presentation of such tests might seem to imply. But, in the absence of more satisfactory techniques, these tests have been used to give some indication of the probability of differences occurring by chance.

Chi-square, t, chi-square trend tests, and tests for differences between proportions have been applied constantly when looking at the data from this survey, and have influenced decisions about what differences to present and how much verbal 'weight' to attach to them. In general, attention has not been drawn to any difference that statistical tests suggest might have occurred by chance five or more times in 100.

Another difficulty about presenting results from a study like this, with over 250 items of basic information from the patients alone, is that of selection. Inevitably not all cross-analyses are carried out – only about 2,000 – and only a fraction of these are presented, which of course gives rise to difficulty in interpreting significance. Positive results are more often shown than negative ones. Readers may sometimes wonder why certain further analyses are not reported. Often, but not always, the analysis will have been done but the result found to be negative or inconclusive.

Table H shows the sampling error for a number of characteristics. (For the appropriate formula see Gray and Corlett (1950).) Because of the wide variations between areas the design effect is relatively large for the proportion of patients with a doctor in a health centre.

Table H Sampling errors

	Mean proportion	*Range in 20 study areas*	*Sampling error*	*Estimated random sampling error**	*Mean ± two sampling errors***	*Design effect ****
Proportion of patients with no general practitioner consultation in previous 12 months	24%	15%–40%	1.9	1.5	20%–28%	1.3
Proportion of patients with an out-patient consultation in previous 12 months	36%	20%–50%	1.9	1.7	32%–40%	1.1
Proportion of patients describing their doctor as 'not so good' about explaining things fully	22%	9%–37%	1.5	1.5	19%–25%	1.0
Proportion of patients with a single-handed doctor	13%	0%–34%	2.2	1.2	9%–17%	1.8
Proportion of patients with a doctor at a health centre	22%	0%–65%	4.2	1.8	14%–30%	2.3

* Of a random sample throughout the country, i.e. $\sqrt{\frac{p \times q}{n}}$

** These have been calculated on precise figures and then rounded off.

*** The ratio of the sampling error with the given two-stage sample design to the estimated random sampling error.

Appendix V
Classification of social class

The classification is based on the classification of occupations (OPCS 1970). This distinguishes six 'social class' groups:

I Professional, etc., occupations

II Intermediate occupations

III Skilled occupations
(N) Non-manual
(M) Manual

IV Partly skilled occupations

V Unskilled occupations.

These classes are intended to reflect 'the general standing within the community of the occupations concerned.' In a number of instances the main differences that emerge are between what can be described as the 'middle class' and 'working class', the former being most of the non-manual occupations – the Registrar General's social classes I, II, and III non-manual – and the latter almost entirely manual – III manual, IV, and V.

Men and single women were classified on the basis of their present occupation if they were under retirement age (65 for men, 60 for women) or on their main occupation if they were over retirement age. Married and widowed women have been classified according to their husband's present or main occupation. This is obviously an unsatisfactory procedure in many ways, partly because women's occupations have very different social class distributions from men's. This can be seen from *Table J*. A high proportion of single women, classified by their own occupations, are classed as skilled non-manual, and therefore as 'middle class'. The class distribution of ever-married women, based on the occupations of their husbands, is similar to that of men.

So by combining these different indices of social class, we are in effect adding chalk to cheese. One consolation is that the proportion of 'chalk', occupations of single women is relatively low, 5%.

Class distributions of our samples in 1964 and 1977 show an increase in the proportion classified as middle class, from 36% in 1964 to 43% in 1977.

Table J Patients' social class by sex and marital status

	Men 1977	*Women 1977*		*All patients 1977*	*All patients 1964*
		Single	*Ever-married*		
Middle class:	%	%	%	%	%
I Professional	8	—	5	6	4
II Intermediate	22	28	21	22	19
III Skilled non-manual	12	49	14	15	13
Working class:					
III Skilled manual	40	7	39	38	40
IV Partly skilled	11	14	15	13	18
V Unskilled	7	2	6	6	6
Number of patients (= 100%)	400	43	362	805	1,341

Appendix VI
Procedures score

This was based on the doctors' responses to the question about whether they personally undertook various procedures in their practice when they arose more often than not, occasionally or never. The procedures were excising simple cysts, taking blood, stitching cuts, and examining vagina with a speculum. Responses are shown in *Table K*.

Table K Action on different procedures

	Excise simple cysts	*Take blood*	*Stitch cuts*	*Examine vagina with speculum*
Personally undertakes procedure in his/her practice:	%	%	%	%
More often than not	29	55	44	83
Occasionally	37	42	43	15
Never	34	3	13	2
Number of doctors (=100%)		362		

Answers to the four questions were combined by scoring two for each procedure they did 'more often than not' and one for the ones they did 'occasionally', giving a maximum of eight and a minimum of nought if they never did any of the procedures. The distribution can be seen in *Table L.*

Table L Distribution of procedures scores

Score	%
0	1
1	1
2	4
3	7
4	14
5	21
6	17
7	14
8	21
Number of doctors (=100%)	362

This indicates that doctors who carried out one procedure were more likely to carry out another, since the expected proportion scoring eight if the procedures were independent is 6%, compared with an observed 21%.

Appendix VII
Private practice and those without a doctor

Four of the five people with private doctors had been dissatisfied with their NHS doctor. Two were critical of the way the doctors had treated their relatives. One said her husband had rung the doctor on a Sunday to ask for some advice about their daughter who had had a recurrence of abscesses in her ears. The doctor had said he did not work on Sundays and had subsequently told them to look for another doctor. The other had asked a doctor to visit her husband who was behaving strangely after a stroke. The doctor on duty had said that if the husband was up he was well enough to go to the surgery. At that point she had contacted a private doctor. Her husband died within a fortnight. The other two criticisms were:

> 'I wasn't satisfied with the treatment he was giving me. It was just a matter of "Take another pill".'

> 'I only went to the NHS doctor once. He couldn't cope with the problem.'

The fifth person with a private doctor said 'English doctors in this area for NHS treatment are impossible to find.' So for all five private medicine had not been their initial preference.

Those without a doctor

All the eleven who were not on the list of an NHS doctor who they would consult if they were ill and did not have a private doctor had been on the list of an NHS doctor in the past. Ten were no longer on an effective list because they had moved or the doctor had moved, retired, or died; the other one had stopped going 'because I don't feel I'm getting any personal attention. They always seem too busy for you.'

Nine of the eleven intended to register with a doctor again. Reasons for not having done so already were mainly that they had not bothered.

'I suppose because it's low on my priorities because I enjoy good health.'

But four of the nine had had some difficulty or inhibition about finding a doctor.

'I have tried – but the one I tried was full up.'

'I've not bothered yet. The days go by and you forget about it. It's knowing where to go.'

'I haven't been sufficiently persistent I suppose and initially I had some trouble in attempting to get on a list.'

'Because I couldn't remember my last doctor's name.'

One who was undecided whether or not to register with an NHS doctor said he did not have time to sit around in waiting rooms. The woman who had stopped going to her doctor because she was unhappy with her treatment was also not sure but said there was not another NHS doctor in her area. When she was on holiday abroad she had been to a doctor.

'He really put the wind up me. He was horrified that I'd been on the pill so long, said I really should be off it now and that I must go and see my doctor when I got back . . . I have to go very soon. I've really decided I suppose that I'm going to (private doctor). But you see I don't think he'd come out here to visit. And if we needed him to come in a hurry . . . I don't know what to say.'

References

ANDERSON, R. (1979) Public Awareness of and Interest in Community Health Councils. *Health and Social Services Journal* **Lxxxix** No 4633.

——(forthcoming) Prescribed medicines: who takes what? *Journal of Epidemiology and Community Health.*

——(In draft) The changes general practitioners would like to see in the NHS.

ARMSTRONG, D. (1979) The Emancipation of Biographical Medicine. *Social Science and Medicine* **13A**: 1–8.

AYLETT, M. J. (1976) Seeing the Same Doctor. *Journal of the Royal College of General Practitioners* **26**: 47–53.

BEALES, J. G. (1978) *Sick Health Centres and How to Make Them Better.* London: Pitman Medical.

BIRMINGHAM RESEARCH UNIT OF THE ROYAL COLLEGE OF GENERAL PRACTITIONERS (1977) Self-evaluation in General Practice. *Journal of the Royal College of General Practitioners* **27**: 265–270.

BONE, M. (1978) *The Family Planning Services: Changes and Effects.* London: HMSO.

BOWLING, A. (forthcoming) *Delegation in General Practice: A Study of Doctors and Nurses.* London: Tavistock.

BRIDGSTOCK, M. (1976) General Practitioners' Organisation and Estimates of their Workload. In *Prescribing in General Practice. Supplement No. 1. Journal of the Royal College of General Practitioners* **26.**

BUCHAN, I. C. and RICHARDSON, I. M. (1973) *Time Study of Consultations in General Practice.* Scottish Health Studies No. 27. Scottish Home and Health Department.

BUTLER, J. R. (1973) *Family Doctors and Public Policy: A Study of Manpower Distribution.* London and Boston: Routledge and Kegan Paul.

CARTWRIGHT, A. (1967) *Patients and Their Doctors.* London: Routledge and Kegan Paul.

——(1970) *Patients and Family Planning Services.* London: Routledge and Kegan Paul.

——(1974) Prescribing and the Relationship Between Patients and Doctors. In, Ruth Cooperstock (ed.) *Social Aspects of the Medical Use of Psychiatric Drugs*. Toronto, Canada. Alcoholism and Drug Addiction Research Foundation of Ontario.

——(1979) *The Dignity of Labour?* London: Tavistock.

CARTWRIGHT, A. and MARSHALL, R. (1965) General Practice in 1963. *Medical Care* **3**: 69–87.

CARTWRIGHT, A. and O'BRIEN, M. (1976) Social Class Variations in Health Care and in the Nature of General Practitioner Consultations. In, Margaret Stacey (ed.) *The Sociology of the NHS*. Sociological review Monograph 22. University of Keele.

CENTRAL STATISTICAL OFFICE (1978) *Social Trends*. London: HMSO.

——(1979) *Social Trends*. London: HMSO.

——(1979) *Annual Abstract of Statistics* London: HMSO.

COUNCIL OF THE ROYAL COLLEGE OF GENERAL PRACTITIONERS (1974) Evidence to the Inquiry into the Regulation of the Medical Profession. *Journal of the Royal College of General Practitioners* **24**: 59–74.

DAWSON REPORT (1920) *Report on the Future Provision of Medical and Allied Services*. London: HMSO.

DEPARTMENT OF HEALTH AND SOCIAL SECURITY (1976) *Priorities for Health and Personal Social Services in England: A Consultative Document*. London: HMSO.

——(1977a) *Annual Report* 1976. London: HMSO.

——(1977b) *Health and Personal Social Services Statistics for England* (with summary tables for Great Britain) 1977. London: HMSO.

——(1978) *Annual Report* 1977. London: HMSO.

DEPARTMENT OF HEALTH AND SOCIAL SECURITY AND WELSH OFFICE (1979) *Patients First*. London: HMSO.

DIXON, R. A. and WILLIAMS, B. T. (1977) Twelve Months of Deputising: 100,000 Patient Contacts with Eighteen Services. *British Medical Journal* **1**: 560–63.

DUNNELL, K. and CARTWRIGHT, A. (1972) *Medicine Takers, Prescribers and Hoarders*. London: Routledge and Kegan Paul.

EARTHROWL, B. and STACEY, M. (1977) Social Class and Children in Hospital. *Social Science and Medicine* **2**: 83–8.

EIMERL, T. S. and PEARSON, R. J. C. (1966) Working Time in General Practice: How General Practitioners Use Their Time. *British Medical Journal* **2**: 1549–554.

FORSYTH, G. and LOGAN, R. F. L. (1960) *The Demand for Medical Care: A Study of the Case-load in the Barrow-in-Furness Group of Hospitals*. London: Oxford University Press.

FOX, T. F. (1960) The Personal Doctor and His Relation to the Hospital. *Lancet* **1**: 743–60.

FREEMAN, J. and BYRNE, P. S. (1973) *The Assessment of Postgraduate Training in General Practice*. Guildford, Surrey. Society for Research into Higher Education.

——(1976) *The Assessment of Vocational Training for General Practice*. Report from General Practice 17 London, *Journal of the Royal College of General Practitioners*.

——(1977) Clinical Factual Recall and Patient Management Skill in General Practice. *Medical Education* **11**: 39–47.

FRY, J. (ed.) (1977) *Trends in General Practice 1977*. London: British Medical Journal.

GARDNER, W. (1979) Absence from Work Attributed to Sickness. In *Management of Minor Illness*. London: King Edward's Hospital Fund for London.

GILCHRIST, I. C. et al. (1978) Social Work in General Practice. *The Journal of the Royal College of General Practitioners* **28**: 675–86.

GOLDBERG, E. M. and NEILL, J. E. (1972) *Social Work in General Practice*. London : George Allen and Unwin.

GRAY, D. J. P. (1978) Feeling at Home. *The Journal of the Royal College of General Practitioners* **28**: 6–17.

GRAY, P. G. and CARTWRIGHT, A. (1953) Choosing and changing Doctors. *Lancet ii* **1**: 308.

GRAY, P. G. and CORLETT, T. (1950) Sampling for the Social Survey. *Journal of the Royal Statistical Society* Series A General **cxiii**: 150–99.

HART, J. T. (1971) The Inverse Care Law. *Lancet* i:405–12.

HARVARD DAVIS REPORT (1971) *The Organisation of Group Practice*. London: HMSO.

HAYNES, S. G., MCMICHAEL, A. J., and TYROLER, H. A. (1977) The Relationship of Normal, Involuntary Retirement to Early Mortality among U.S. Rubber Workers. *Social Science and Medicine* **11**: 105–14.

HICKS, D. (1976) *Primary Health Care*. London: HMSO.

HONIGSBAUM, F. (1979) *The Division in British Medicine*. London: Kogan Page.

HORDER, J. P. (1977) Physicians and Family Doctors: a New Relationship. *Journal of the Royal College of General Practitioners* **27**: 391–97.

HOWIE, J. (1977) *Patterns of Work*. In John Fry (ed.) *Trends in General Practice 1977*. London, for the Royal College of General Practitioners by the British Medical Journal.

IRVINE, D. and JEFFERYS, M. (1971) BMA Planning Unit Survey of General Practice 1969. *British Medical Journal* **4**: 535–43.

JEFFERYS, M. (1976) Foreword to *Team Care in General Practice* by Geoffrey Marsh and Peter Kaim-Caudle. London : Croom Helm.

Journal of the Royal College of General Practitioners (1979) Editorial **29**: 67–8.

LEEUWENHORST WORKING PARTY (1977) *Journal of the Royal College of General Practitioners* **27**: 117.

LOGAN, W. P. D. and CUSHION, A. A. (1958) *Morbidity Statistics from General Practice. Vol. 1 (General)*. Studies on Medical and Population Subjects No. 14. London: HMSO.

MCCORMICK, J. (1979) *The Doctor: Father Figure or Plumber*. London: Croom Helm.

MARINKER, M. (1974) Medical Education and Human Values. *Journal of the Royal College of General Practitioners* **24**: 445–62.

MARSH, G. M. (1977) 'Curing' Minor Illness in General Practice. *British Medical Journal* **2**: 1267–269.

MARSH, G. and KAIM-CAUDLE, P. (1976) *Team Care in General Practice.* London: Croom Helm.

MINISTRY OF HEALTH (1965) *Annual Report of the Ministry of Health for the Year 1964.* London: HMSO.

MORGAN, W., WALKER, J. H., HOLOHAN, A. M., and RUSSELL, I. T. (1974) Casual Attenders: a Socio-Medical Study of Patients attending Accident and Emergency Departments in the Newcastle upon Tyne Area. *Hospital and Health Services Review,* June 1974: 189–194.

NORELL, J. S. Personal communication.

OFFICE OF POPULATION CENSUSES AND SURVEYS (1970) Classification of Occupations 1970. London: HMSO.

——(1978a) *Demographic Review 1977.* London: HMSO.

——(1978b) *Electoral Statistics.* London: HMSO.

OFFICE OF POPULATION CENSUSES AND SURVEYS, SOCIAL SURVEY DIVISION (1973–1979) *The General Household Survey.* London: HMSO.

PETERSON, O. L., ANDREWS, L. P., SPAIN, R. S., and GREENBERG, B. G. (1956) An Analytic Study of North Carolina General Practice 1953–54. *Journal of Medical Education* **31**: 1 (No. 12 Part 2).

REEDY, B. L. E. C. (1977) The Health Team. In, John Fry (ed.) *Trends in General Practice 1977* London, for the Royal College of General Practitioners by the British Medical Journal.

REEDY, B. L. E. C., PHILIPS, P. R., and NEWELL, D. J. (1976) Nurses and Nursing in Primary Medical Care in England. *British Medical Journal* **2**: 1304.

REID, I. (1977) *Social Class Differences in Britain.* London: Open Books.

REVIEW BODY ON DOCTORS' AND DENTISTS' REMUNERATION (1977) *Seventh report.* London: HMSO.

RITCHIE, J., JACOBY, A. and BONE, M. (1980) *Access to Primary Health Care.* London: HMSO.

ROYAL COLLEGE OF GENERAL PRACTITIONERS (1972) *The Future General Practitioner – Learning and Teaching.* London: British Medical Journal.

——(1974a) *Morbidity Statistics from General Practice. Second National Study 1970–71.* Studies on Medical and Population Subjects No. 26 London: HMSO.

——(1974b) *The General Practitioner in Europe.* A statement by the Working Party appointed by the Second European Conference on the Teaching of General Practice. Leeuwenhorst Netherlands.

ROYAL COMMISSION ON MEDICAL EDUCATION (1978) (Todd). London: HMSO.

ROYAL COMMISSION ON THE NATIONAL HEALTH SERVICE (1979) (Merrison). London: HMSO.

SMITH, C. (1981) How Complete is the Electoral Register? *Political Studies.*

SMITH, D. J. (1980) *Overseas Doctors in the National Health Service.* London: Heinemann.

SOWERBY, P. (1977) The Doctor, his Patient, and the Illness: a Reappraisal. *Journal of the Royal College of General Practitioners* **27**: 583–89.

STEVENS, J. L. (1977) Quality of Care in General Practice: Can it be Assessed? *Journal of the Royal College of General Practitioners*. **27**: 455–66.

STEVENSON, J. S. K. (1967) Appointment Systems in General Practice: How Patients use Them. *British Medical Journal* **2**: 827–29.

STIMSON, G. and WEBB, B. (1975) *Going to See the Doctor*. London and Boston: Routledge and Kegan Paul.

THOMAS, K. B. (1978) The Consultation and the Therapeutic Illusion. *British Medical Journal* **1**: 1327–328.

U.S. DEPARTMENT OF HEALTH, EDUCATION AND WELFARE (1972). Age Patterns in Medical Care, Illness and Disability. United States, 1968–1969. Washington. *Vital and Health Statistics*. Data from the National Health Survey Series 10, No. 70.

VERBRUGGE, L. M. (1979) Female Illness Rates and Illness Behaviour. *Women and Health* **4**: 61–79.

WATKIN, B. (1975) *Documents on Health and Social Services 1834 to the Present Day*. London: Methuen.

WILLIAMS, P. and CLARE, A. (1979) Social Workers in Primary Health Care: the General Practitioner's Viewpoint. *Journal of the Royal College of General Practitioners* **29**: 554–58.

WILLIAMS, W. O. (1970) *Study of General Practitioners' Workload in South Wales 1965–1966*. Royal College of General Practitioners. Reports from General Practice No. 12.

WOFINDEN, R. C. (1967) Health Centres and the General Medical Practitioner. *British Medical Journal* **2**: 565–67.

WOLFE, S. and BADGELY, R. F. (1974) How Much is Enough? The Payment of Doctors – Implications for Health Policy in Canada. *International Journal of Health Services* **4** (2): 245–64.

Name index

Subject index